The Best American Medical Writing 2009

Foreword by
Pauline W. Chen, MD

KAPLAN)

PUBLISHING

New York

This publication is designed to provide accurate and authoritative information in regard to the subject matter covered. It is sold with the understanding that the publisher is not engaged in rendering legal, accounting, or other professional service. If legal advice or other expert assistance is required, the services of a competent professional should be sought.

Published by Kaplan Publishing, a division of Kaplan, Inc.
1 Liberty Plaza, 24th Floor
New York, NY 10006

ISBN-13: 978-1-60714-464-9

Kaplan Publishing books are available at special quantity discounts to use for sales promotions, employee premiums, or educational purposes. Please email our Special Sales Department to order or for more information at *kaplanpublishing@kaplan.com*, or write to Kaplan Publishing, 1 Liberty Plaza, 24th Floor, New York, NY 10006.

Table of Contents

Introduction

Pauline W. Chen

From the age of seven until the year I started medical school, I played the violin. Though never prodigiously talented, I eventually became proficient enough to make a few extra dollars teaching beginners during my last two years of high school.

The method I used to teach was the one I had used to learn: the Suzuki method. Just as babies learn language, Suzuki students learn to play, listening repeatedly to songs they will later "mimic" on their instruments. The results of this pedagogical approach can be astounding. I have seen three-year-olds who can barely describe what they are doing play "Twinkle, Twinkle" flawlessly on their downsized instruments.

The key to the method's success, at least in my experience, is not acquiring the mechanics of playing the violin. It is all that listening—folk songs, Bach, Vivaldi, the great classical pieces selected by Mr. Shinichi Suzuki himself. Mr. Suzuki understood one thing well—that hearing a song over and over again does more than imprint it in your memory; it etches the language of music in your soul.

A grace note inserted at the right point lightens the musical line; a series of staccatos speeds it up. Several grand chords in a row signal an impending ending, the drama of which turns precisely on the number of chords used. Too many chords result in music that feels amateurish or overwrought; too few leave the listener feeling cheated. Patterns of musical phrasing and cadence come to hold meaning that can, in turn, reliably evoke a range of emotion.

I rarely pull out my fiddle now. But I still find myself endlessly thinking about musical sounds, particularly when I write. In my mind, I listen over and over again to the words in a sentence or paragraph, tweaking them until their sounds and meaning not only evoke the ideas I am trying to convey but also fit comfortably into those musical motifs etched in my soul.

And consciously or not, I rely on that databank of musical patterns every time I read. The best writing possesses a musicality so fundamental, so natural, that it is no longer discernible. Like some primal biochemical reaction, the sounds on the page slide into their respective receptors within the mind, triggering a surge of emotion. Writing that does so perfectly is writing that goes straight to my heart, locking in perfectly into the pattern set there years ago by Mr. Suzuki.

IT COMES AS no surprise, then, that I fell back on my musical training as I read through the pieces carefully culled together by my editor, Matthew Laird. But before choosing the pieces for this inaugural edition of *Best American Medical Writing*, there were two issues that needed to be resolved.

First, what is *medical* writing?

Most people would agree that medicine involves healthcare, illness, caregiving, science, and wellness. Medical writing, it would naturally follow, is writing that touches on any of those topics. But the definition I finally came to use, my definition of *best* medical writing, involves more than writing, let's say, about cancer, healthcare costs, DNA snippets, or anterior cruciate ligament injuries. The best medical writing illuminates the vulnerability that comes with having a body, with being human.

Regardless of whether we are clinicians or lay people, our bodies will, eventually, fail us. That failure may come in the form of an acute traumatic injury, a lifelong struggle with a chronic illness, or the occasional cold. Whatever the manifestation, once sick we will find ourselves navigating the healthcare system, depending on caregivers, looking toward science for understanding and help, and seeking ways to feel and remain well. All of those experiences are medicine; but none of them, as anyone who has ever ignored crushing substernal chest pain can attest, will necessarily pin you down and force you to reflect on your essential humanity. The best medical writing does.

The second issue that needed to be resolved had to do with the form of writing. Medicine lends itself to one of the most expansive literary canvases, ranging from the most delicate of poetic stanzas to the densest of peer-reviewed journal articles. For me, the possibility of including all those forms of writing in this collection was intoxicating; the reality of it was overwhelming.

In the end, I decided that I would focus primarily on essays. Essays are easily understood by clinicians and non-clinicians alike, and they are the literary form that I have always found most resembles clinical thinking—a seamless blend of science and art with good doses of personal reflection. Moreover, essays have a kind of elasticity about them; they can encompass all the messy, complicated, gritty, sometimes humorous, often opaque, and always personal experiences that make up medicine without ever losing their essential narrative form.

While there is a long tradition of physicians writing about medicine, nearly half of this collection is made up of essays written by patients or the family caregivers of those patients who cannot speak for themselves. There is a well-known aphorism in clinical medicine: Insight into any diagnostic dilemma can be readily found in the patient's story. The same could be said for medical writing. Some of the essays in this group are irreverent, others are angry, and a few are even laugh-out-loud funny. But whatever the voice, each illuminates a unique aspect of the experience of being ill, of facing down one's own vulnerability.

Dana Jennings, in "Real Men Get Prostate Cancer," shatters the silence on topics too often ignored or glossed over in discussions between patients with prostate cancer and their families and clinicians. Jennings describes being diagnosed with prostate cancer and his treatment with Lupron, a form of hormone therapy that reduces testosterone to castration levels. With humor, dignity, and great honesty, he writes about the effects of the treatment on his sex drive, his sense of masculinity, and his relationship with his wife and family, topics that "shake the very pillars of what we talk about when we talk about being a man."

In "I Want My Life Back," Andrea Coller, a 27-year-old woman, describes being diagnosed with recurrent cancer. With a series of one-sentence paragraphs that feel more like poetry than essay, Coller unsparingly describes waking up from a coma in the intensive care unit with a breathing tube in her mouth, navigating well-meaning but thoughtless comments from others, and spitting up the blood that is the calling card of her tumor's return. Every one of her sentences shimmers with life, so much so you cannot help believing—and hoping—that she will write more.

Three of the essays give voice to the difficult task of caregiving. Kevin Baker, in "Mind Bomb," writes about a modern medical nightmare that no caregiver ever wants to face: caring for the ailing parent who, through a genetic roll of the dice, may be a mirror of your own future. Baker lovingly describes his mother's inexorable deterioration from an inherited neurodegenerative disease; but when he discovers that there is a test available for the responsible gene, he must ask himself if he really wants to know.

In one of the most moving pieces in the collection, "Caregiving: The Odyssey of Becoming More Human," Arthur Kleinman writes of caring for his ailing wife, his "intellectual, aesthetic, sexual, emotional, moral" partner of 43 years. It is an existence of "enduring the unendurable." But his descriptions of their most routine interactions—his dressing her, his feeding her—are suffused with such tender intimacy that Kleinman hardly needs to articulate, as he later does, his essay's point: that we become more human by cultivating ourselves and our relationships with others.

Grace Talusan, in "Blinded," writes about her beloved two-year-old niece who has been diagnosed with a retinoblastoma, an eye tumor. The first time I read Talusan's essay, I began crying in the middle of a bookstore café; many reads later, her words still squeeze my heart. As we discover in her piece, Talusan's father, the child's grandfather, is a highly respected ophthalmologist, but, as Talusan writes in prose that is made all the more powerful by its sparseness, "love obstructed my father's vision." His missed diagnosis of his granddaughter's tumor may carry devastating physical, as well as emotional, consequences.

Oliver Sacks is neither a patient with bipolar disorder nor a caregiver, but he manages to create trenchant descriptions of both points of view in "A Summer of Madness." Pulling threads from some of the most important historical and modern works on manic-depression, Sacks weaves a vivid tableau while reviewing *Hurry Down Sunshine,* Michael Greenberg's memoir about his daughter's struggle with bipolar disease. Sacks' review is filled with pitch perfect descriptions of the "cauldronous, fluctuating nature" of the disease and of the exhausting state of hypervigilance that besets family caregivers. The result is a portrayal that does far more than inform; it "remind[s] us of what a narrow ridge of normality we all inhabit, with the abysses of mania and depression yawning to either side."

Caregivers are often called upon to help patients navigate the minefield that is the healthcare system. The experience can be akin to entering an alternate reality, even for the most savvy among us. Two essays describe that reality in strikingly different but equally affecting ways. In "My Daughter's $29,000 Appendectomy," an essay that had me in turns cringing in empathy and laughing out loud (on a small commuter plane, no less), Tom McGrath tracks down the who, what, where, why, and how of his daughter's hospital bills. But as he attempts to disentangle what he terms the "Gordian knot" of healthcare financing, he manages to uncover the fundamental flaw of our healthcare system, one that has prevented and may continue to prevent us from effectively reining in costs.

More haunting in tone is Harold Pollack's recount, "Lessons from an Emergency Room Nightmare." Pollack, a national expert on health administration and director of the University of

Chicago's Center for Health Administration Studies, writes about his wife suddenly developing chest pain and needing emergency treatment. Despite all of his expertise, his wife's experience is bewildering and riddled with missteps. After all is said and done, Pollack reflects on the kind of systemic changes that must occur to prevent similar errors from ever occurring; and it is with poignant regret that Pollack accepts responsibility for the mistakes he has made and forgives those made by others.

Several of the essays come from clinicians themselves. The act of caring for others, even in a purely professional setting, has the power to transform an individual profoundly. Theresa Brown, a former English professor recently turned nurse, describes a patient's death in "Perhaps Death is Proud; More Reason to Savor Life." Brown finds the event unsettling, and she reflects upon several disconnects in her new life. There is the discrepancy between the clinicians' intentions to cure and the constant presence of death, the disparity between the sanitized media images of dying and the "flesh-eating zombie" cadaver before her. What she ultimately takes away from this patient's death has little to do with those poetic romantic notions she once taught; rather they are practical lessons for living that we would all do well to learn.

In "The Moral of the Story," Perri Klass, a pediatrician, describes seeing a 20-month-old boy with a young doctor-in-training. She sends the patient home with antibiotics and Tylenol but that night is haunted by doubts regarding her diagnosis. In this essay, Klass gives voice to the unsettling "what-ifs" that plague every conscientious doctor and describes, with as lyrical a cadence as I've ever seen, the "collective medical memory" of our profession, the stories and experiences that connect in our mind doctors to other doctors, doctors to patients, and patients to other patients.

Two of the essays by clinicians describe the changing demographics of health care professionals in this country. International Medical Graduates, or IMGs, now comprise roughly a quarter of all physicians practicing in the U.S. In "Disorientation," Alok A. Khorana writes about his experiences as an IMG, beginning with his work in a dilapidated two-story public ward in India, followed by the terrifying first night on call in a New York academic medical center. Throughout his essay, Khorana subtly sheds light on the cultural assumptions that are imbued in even the smallest details of patient care.

The demographics of gender continue to change as well. Women now make up more than half of all entering classes in medical school, but, as Julie R. Rosenbaum skillfully describes in "Duality," combining academic practice with the demands of family remains challenging. Using a split-voice narrative, Rosenbaum juxtaposes a profession-wide examination of parental leave policies, job flexibility and promotions with the details of her typical Monday—the needs of two young children, one of whom is may be harboring an infection; a husband working out-of-town; a patient who requires more attention just as she needs to pick up her children from daycare. By the end of the essay—and Rosenbaum's exhausting day—it is more than clear that better workplace policies are not only fair but also long overdue.

While medicine and medical writing have traditionally focused on the patient, the frailty of the body extends to clinicians as well. One of the first pieces I read for this collection was David France's "Another AIDS Casualty." France reflects on the meteoric rise and the equally fast free-fall downward of Dr. Ramon Torres, one of the first physicians to devote his career to AIDS patients. The journey is terrifying, in part because Torres' vulnerability is one that we all share. France quotes playwright and activist Larry Kramer: "If you're a doctor in the midst of all of that, and you've got hundreds of patients, and every one of them is facing death and is terrified, of course you're going to crack up. You wouldn't be a human being if you didn't."

Jason Zengerle, in "Going Under," writes about Dr. Brent Cambron, a rising superstar anesthesiologist who becomes hopelessly addicted to the very medications he administers to others. In recounting this tale, Zengerle brings to life the intractability and equally opportunistic nature of the rising problem of drug addiction among anesthesiologists. The very act of caring for others, controlling someone else's body, may be a catalyst for addiction. As one anesthesiologist quips, " . . . I think that creates a false sense that if we can control what's going on with somebody else, we should be able to control this in ourselves."

Among all the essays, there were two news features stories that I included in the collection because both revealed how healthcare can inspire extraordinary courage and selflessness. Diane Suchetka's "Fixing Mr. Fix-It" was a six-part series that appeared in the *Cleveland Plain Dealer*. Norman Martin, a Cleveland mechanic, is involved in a devastating accident—both of his arms are traumatically amputated when the hydraulic lift holding a 35-ton firetruck above him fails. Suchetka follows Martin for close to a year as he goes through surgery and rehabilitation, skillfully weaving in the multiple personages involved in Martin's care. The end effect is a moving snapshot of healthcare, and people, at their very best.

In "Doctors Within Borders," Susanna Schrobsdorff writes about the work done by volunteer doctors, dentists, nurses, and assistants for Remote Area Medical, a non-profit organization that provides basic medical and dental care in inaccessible areas throughout the world. Schrobsdorff describes one RAM event along the Kentucky border, a region where poverty, poor knowledge about dental care and nutrition, and lack of healthcare access result in one of the highest rates of tooth loss in the United States. Over the course of two and a half days, the RAM event, involving some 1,800 volunteer clinicians and assistants, ends up serving roughly 2,500 patients. For free.

No collection on medical writing would be complete without essays devoted to the kind of humble sleuthing that goes on in laboratories, hospitals, and fields. In "Contagious Cancer," David Quammen writes about the strange phenomenon of tumor contagion between Tasmanian devils, the piglet-sized marsupials that make their home on the Australian island-state of Tasmania. Quammen describes the painstaking work of veterinarians who first notice the lethal, disfiguring facial tumors and then attempt to understand them. In telling his story, Quammen draws upon multiple theories of tumor development and transmission. He links the devils' experience to that of humans, recounting cases of contagious human cancers, tumors that occurred because of surgical implantation, needle sticks, scalpel cuts, and transplantation.

Jessica Snyder Sachs, in "DNA Pollution May be Spawning Killer Microbes," writes about scientists who are investigating DNA pollution. The work is painstaking, but Sachs perfectly captures the idealism that drives these scientists' work. Combing through soil, water, and sewage, they isolate snippets of rogue genetic material, some of which can confer the kind of drug resistance that has been implicated in some 90,000 potentially fatal infections each year in the United States.

Finally, several of the essays in this collection take on the metaphor of war to illustrate some of the most challenging quandaries in modern healthcare. Medicine is often cast as a battle, as a struggle between the individual and the illness, the disease and the therapy, or the afflicted and the unafflicted. The analogy is made even more powerful when it is used, as these essays use it, to explore our assumptions and our inherent vulnerability in these battles. Sharon Begley, in "We Fought Cancer . . . And Cancer Won," turns the metaphor on its head and in the process writes what is perhaps the finest telling of the "war on cancer" I have ever read. She eloquently catalogues the challenges of cancer research and treatment, among them the use of an animal model that poorly mimics the human disease state, and throws light on the pivotal role of private donations in a funding environment that is peer-reviewed but extremely risk-averse.

In "America's AIDS Apartheid," Kai Wright shows us how early therapeutic successes and our subsequent focus on the international front of AIDS have resulted in unparalleled devastation right in our own backyard. The South has become the "new ground zero for America's AIDS epidemic," writes Wright, accounting for more than half of all new U.S. infections between 2001 and 2004. Moreover, these infections were more likely to affect those who were low-income African Americans without the resources necessary to take advantage of the $20,000 per year price tag for protease inhibitors.

In "Virtual Iraq," Sue Halpern writes about using virtual reality to treat Post-Traumatic Stress Disorder, or PTSD, a disorder said to affect at least 17 percent of soldiers returning from Iraq. Halpern describes the desensitization process and manages to capture the eclectic personalities that have driven this unorthodox approach ("an unholy alliance between academia, Hollywood, and the military," states the computer program's inventor).

Michael Sokolove's "The Uneven Playing Field" underscores the struggle between social mores and the body. In the wake of Title IX, the rising numbers of girls participating in sports, and increasing pressures to succeed, an unprecedented number of high school girls have suffered from severe knee injuries. Sokolove weaves the individual and social threads of this tale, casting light on a "perfect storm" that may leave large numbers of women in the future permanently disabled by injuries sustained during their youth.

And lastly, Jerome Groopman's "Superbugs" is about the increasing prevalence of resistant bacteria in hospitals and the community. Written like a great war story, Groopman explores how both sides—humans and bugs—are driven to survive and describes the complex strategies they each employ. But the siren call of antibiotics proves over and over again to be too alluring; we humans cannot help but prescribe them for ourselves and our livestock. In the end, Groopman shows us, we are our own worst enemies. As in many of the lost battles of medicine, we lack the self-awareness, the fundamental understanding of our own weaknesses, to make our lives better.

But great medical writing, like the essays in this volume, can change that.

The Moral of the Story

Perri Klass, MD

From the *New England Journal of Medicine*

I CAME HOME the other night clutching a scrap of paper towel with a mother's cell-phone number scribbled on it. I had been precepting in the residents' pediatric primary care clinic, and an intern had presented a patient: a 20month-old boy who had been brought in by his mother because he was vomiting. He'd thrown up seven times since 2 that morning. No diarrhea, but he wasn't eating or drinking much. Still, he didn't look dehydrated, his mother said he'd had several wet diapers, and when the intern examined him, she found his diaper wet again.

The intern said he had a temperature of 100.8°F, and his ears looked infected. "Oh, great," I said, "so we know what's going on."

She nodded but looked puzzled. "Why would an ear infection make him throw up?" she asked hesitantly.

When I answered honestly—some kids have touchy stomachs, and when they get sick with anything, they throw up—she looked disappointed; she was expecting

pathophysiology. I drew myself up. Perhaps, I suggested, the ear infection was the sequela of a preexisting upper respiratory infection, and the child was producing a lot of mucus, which was dripping into the stomach and provoking the emesis. That went over a little better.

We went in to see the child. He was a sweet, clingy toddler, warily sheltering on his mother's shoulder, and he didn't look happy to see me. In fact, he started crying, which allowed me to verify that indeed he was not dehydrated, since his face was soon wet with tears. I examined him and agreed that his ears looked infected, the eardrums red on both sides and one of them bulging, not moving, hinting at infected fluid behind it. Yes, I said, good job, I agree, not dangerously dehydrated, I agree, ear infection. And let's remind the mother to encourage him to drink liquids and watch him carefully to make sure he doesn't get dehydrated. I smiled at the mother reassuringly and was relieved to see that she looked mature and competent, as she comforted and soothed her child with efficient, fond caresses.

But she looked anxious. She had something else she wanted to bring up, something she hadn't told the intern or mentioned to me when I was questioning her. "Doctor, let me ask you one more thing," she said. "It couldn't be that this was from falling down, could it? From falling down the stairs?"

And out came the story: the night before last, the child's brother had come up the stairs from the basement, and when he opened the door, the baby was right there, reaching for something, and he fell forward down the stairs. "I didn't see it," she said, "but I heard the thump-thump-thump when he fell. And his brother said he got hurt all over his head. But that couldn't be doing this, right?"

So we had a problem. One of the danger signs after head trauma is vomiting. Here was a child who had fallen down a flight of stairs about a day and a half ago and a little more than 24 hours later had begun throwing up repeatedly.

And I was about to send him home with a diagnosis of acute otitis media.

I could see that I was disappointing the mother when I didn't just wave it away: don't be silly, what could one thing have to do with the other? She had offered up the falling-down-the-stairs story as a "doorknob moment"—the doctor essentially done, her hand (or the patient's) literally or figuratively on the doorknob, and the patient brings up a deliberately by-the-way question that turns the whole thing inside out. So I put her through the story in more detail, and it sounded pretty benign: just a few wooden steps, the whole flight maybe 3 feet high. The child hadn't been knocked out—a sign that the head trauma was relatively minor. The mother hadn't noticed any changes in how he was walking—though actually, he wasn't walking much; he was too clingy because he was feeling sick. Of course, he didn't have the language to say whether he felt pain. And even if he'd had language, he could have pointed at his head and told us it hurt and left us completely unsure whether it was his head or his ear.

Head trauma shouldn't give you even a low-grade fever, I told myself. The time course of the emesis wasn't textbook—it had started more than 24 hours after the fall, and it seemed to have resolved after a few hours. And the child looked good, didn't he? Well, he was clearly not dehydrated, which had loomed as the major danger when I walked into the room. But could I go further than that? The words I would have used to describe him were clingy and cranky—words deliberately chosen, in part, because they don't sound medical alarms. Clingy and cranky, not playful or active; in fact, he was unwilling to walk. I asked his mother to put him down for a minute, but when she tried, he began to wail. He pulled up his legs into the fetal position, and goodbye to any hope of assessing his gait to confirm that he looked neurologically normal. It's like that with toddlers. His mother smiled at me apologetically as she gathered him up again. "He's been like this," she said. "Not running around. Not playing so much."

We examined his head for bumps or bruises. We went over the story again. Finally, I sent the mother home with prescriptions for amoxicillin and acetaminophen and gave her some of the what-towatch-for signs off the standard head-trauma information sheet: if he starts vomiting again, if he seems less alert than usual, come to the emergency room. I wrote her phone number on a piece of paper towel, saying I'd call her later to see how he was doing.

And I worried. It would be silly to send him to the emergency room or radiology when the overwhelming odds were that he just had an ear infection. The timing didn't really make sense for a head bleed, I told myself, and he looked like a kid with a viral syndrome.

Later that night, when I called, the mother was as reassuring as could be: "Oh, Doctor, he's doing great, he's playing, he's running around, he's really acting like himself. He even ate a little bit." No more emesis, no mental-status changes, normal energy level restored.

But I've been thinking ever since about why I was so worried. It's not such an unusual story, after all, a toddler who took a fall. I've probably examined dozens of children who were brought in with that as the chief complaint: fell off the bed, tumbled out of the stroller, climbed up on the back of the couch and dived right over. I've felt their heads and looked in their eyes. Some I've sent to radiology, but not most. Some I've worried about for obvious reasons—concerns about child abuse and inflicted injury—and I've looked them over for bruises and unexplained marks. Some I've sent home with their parents holding head-trauma instruction sheets. And so far, nothing terrible has transpired with any of them.

So why did this boy get me so worried? Maybe precisely because the head trauma wasn't the reason for the visit. He was brought in for vomiting, and we didn't even think to ask about head trauma, because the vomiting seemed to be part of some viral syndrome, and we heard about it only in the elaborately casual doorknob question. Somehow that made it seem much more likely that the injury was severe, the story not what it appeared to be. I hadn't asked the right question, I had been pursuing the wrong story. I had almost missed this history altogether—didn't that make it more likely that I'd missed something serious?

Wouldn't that turn out to be the "teaching point" if you were telling this story to medical students? Listen properly, and don't overtake the patient's narrative with your own, or you'll miss the most important information. And if I listened properly and rephrased the story as that of a 20-monthold with a history of emesis times seven and recent head trauma from a fall down the stairs, didn't that sound kind of serious?

Somehow, this encounter had tripped a wire with me—a wire braided, I realized, of history and literature. The literature was the Raymond Carver story "A Small, Good Thing," about a child who is hit by a car, who "got unsteadily to his feet. The boy wobbled a little. He looked dazed, but okay." He walks home and tells his mother, and then he becomes unconscious. The story traces his hospital course and describes the nightmare days and nights of his parents' vigil and the doctors' well-meaning but inept attempts to communicate with the parents and ultimately futile efforts to save the child. It's a hard story for a parent or a pediatrician to read.

There's a moment in it when the child has just been hospitalized, newly unconscious. The doctor has spoken to the parents in highly reassuring terms, and the boy's father decides to go home and bathe and change his clothes.

Howard drove home from the hospital. He took the wet, dark streets very fast, then caught himself and slowed down.

Until now, his life had gone smoothly and to his satisfaction—
college, marriage, another year of college for the advanced
degree in business, a junior partnership in an investment firm.
Fatherhood. He was happy and, so far, lucky—he knew that. . .
So far, he had kept away from any real harm, from those forces
he knew existed and that could cripple or bring down a man if
the luck went bad, if things suddenly turned.

There it is, I thought, rereading the story. The understanding of how close we all are to being unlucky. The child who
steps off a curb without looking. The story in the exam room
that you don't listen to properly. The superficially well patient
who is sicker than anyone thinks. So I had this story stuck in
my mind, and the message I remembered best is one Carver
probably never intended, one better suited to an ER instruction
sheet: Even minor head trauma can be serious.

At the same time, I had a true story nagging at me, one that
my own preceptor in primary care told when I was a pediatric
resident. We had been talking about head injuries, and the preceptor had offered up a grim story: an adolescent who had hit
his head in some freak accident but seemed fine and then died
from an unsuspected bleed. The story had made a tremendous
impression on me—because what sounded like a minor injury
had killed someone, because it had happened in the practice
of a very good doctor whom I regarded as my mentor, because
he knew the family well and had been the one they called when
their son died.

But I had heard that story at least 20 years earlier, when it
was already many years old, and I wondered how much of it I was
inventing. So I tracked down my preceptor and called him and
said, rather hesitantly, "I think there was a story you told, back in
1986 or 1987, and it's stayed with me all these years. Something
about head trauma that sounded minor but wasn't?"

"I know exactly what you mean," he said. "It broke my
heart." And he told the story again: "A 10-year-old boy sliding

off the iced roofs of cars in a parking lot, he fell and struck his head. It was relatively minor, he was brought to an emergency room, was examined, had skull films. That was the standard then, before the days of readily available CTs. . . I was off that weekend. The mom called me on Monday to say he had a bit of a headache but he was okay. Not vomiting, not great, but he was okay. I presumed he had a post-concussion headache. And then at 2 in the morning, I had a call from the mom that he'd stopped breathing and he'd been brought by ambulance to an emergency room some distance off and they were resuscitating him. So I jumped in the car at 2 A.M., and off I went to this place, in time to pronounce him dead." He paused. "He was a sweet boy, a good boy."

And then—once your preceptor, always your preceptor—he took me through the story of the child I had seen in clinic and agreed with the management. "But I thought about your story," I said. "I guess I always think about your story a little bit, and this time I really thought about it."

"The moral of the story is that minor head injuries are significant," he said. "It still grieves me—I must have been full of sadness when I discussed it with the group. But over the course of my 30-plus years, this little boy who died is the only one."

"So what is the real moral?" I asked.

"Medicine is knowledge, judgment, experience, and luck," he said.

So I have been thinking about the voices that echo in your head when you make a clinical decision—even a relatively low-acuity decision about a child who doesn't seem critically ill. You can't let all the what-ifs terrorize you, or you would do a lumbar puncture on every young child with a high fever and do a CT scan for even the most minor bump on the head. So you just go on practicing, haunted by stories—stories you're a part of, stories that happen to people you love or know well or take care of, stories you hear from your teachers and colleagues, and the occasional well-told story that enters your brain and lives there

. . . all those ghosts that hover at your shoulder or in the dark places of your mind. I had a peculiar sense of multiple levels of precepting—of me standing over the intern, and my preceptor standing over me, and of the ways that your medical education comes down to you partly from people you will never meet.

I'd like to think of it, in part, as a collective medical memory. And also as a way of honoring the patients who have suffered "bad outcomes"—and their physicians, too, the ones who are grieving still, who have told and retold these difficult stories. Bad things can be only a step away, and we need to absorb that knowledge and yet still do our job. It seems to me right and proper that even in everyday primary care, there should arise these unexpected, unpredictable moments when the collective memory catches at your sleeve, when the ghosts whisper to you to watch out, to think again, or at least to scribble a cell-phone number on a piece of paper towel and call later just to be sure that everything's truly okay.

No potential conflict of interest relevant to this article was reported.

My Daughter's $29,000 Appendectomy

Tom McGrath

From *Philadelphia Magazine*

When the bills and insurance forms for my five-year-old's surgery started rolling in, I was the one who needed a doctor. So I set out on a quest to understand them—and learned just how screwed up our health-care system really is.

IT BEGAN THE way these things often begin.

"Sarah threw up in the car!" my daughter Hannah announced brightly one evening as she and her sister got home from the performing-arts class they were taking. Hannah is in third grade and three years older than her kindergarten-age sister, but the mythic status of the Kid Who Pukes In An Inappropriate Place transcends time, space and age gap. I know this not only because of my daughters, but because it has been 35 years since I was in third grade, and I can still conjure up both the names of the kids who heaved in our grade-school hallway *and* what it smelled like. (Hope you're feeling better, Linda U.)

My wife Kate and I figured that our usually spirited five-year-old was suffering from a run-of-the-mill stomach bug, so over the course of the next day and a half, Kate did what she does so well: gave Sarah lots of TLC, read to her, played with her, watched Barbie DVDs with her. By Saturday morning, Sarah was feeling better—or at least I thought she *should* be feeling better, which is why, in a decision that will undoubtedly be part of my father-of-the-year nomination, I announced that Sarah should walk with me to an event at Hannah's school, a short distance from our house.

"But my tummy hurts," Sarah whimpered, still in the prone position she had taken up on our living room couch.

"Sarah," I began, dropping into my deep "I am your father therefore I am very wise therefore you would do well to heed me" voice, "you probably just have a little gas. Taking a walk will actually make your tummy feel better."

Within a couple of blocks, it was clear that Sarah's "gas" wasn't going anywhere. "It *hurts*," she wailed, doubling over in front of a neighbor's house. So I finally relented and told her that if she insisted on acting like a *little girl* about this, fine, we didn't have to go to Hannah's school.

Then, naturally, I made her walk home.

As the hours passed, Sarah didn't get better; she got worse. By five o'clock, my wife was on the phone with our pediatrician. Standing in the kitchen, I listened as she described Sarah's circumstances—she left out the kindergarten version of the Bataan Death March I'd led my daughter on—and nodded before hanging up.

"He says we have to go to the hospital—*now*," Kate said. "It's probably her appendix."

I'll spare you any more suspense. At 3 A.M. the next morning, nine hours after we'd arrived at the emergency room at Children's Hospital of Philadelphia, after various exams, X-rays, ultrasounds and IVs, a very cool surgeon named Peter Mattei made three tiny incisions in my daughter's belly and slid out her minute, misbehaving appendix. Over the next couple of days, with the help of my wife, who never left her side, and a team of wonderful doctors and nurses, Sarah recovered the way most surgical patients recover: a good hour here, a bad one there, a burst of energy here, a three-hour coma-like nap there. On Tuesday afternoon, three days after we'd rushed her to the hospital, Sarah came home—lacking one appendix, but having gained two Webkinz stuffed animals, which made her older sister jealous enough that she was clearly trying to figure out how *she* could land in the hospital.

On one level, I—and, I think, my wife—look at Sarah's appendectomy as something of a miracle. In the broadest possible terms, something went haywire in the belly of our little girl, and over the course of several days, dozens—and I mean dozens—of highly trained, highly capable people worked together to fix it. They did such a remarkable job that within a week of coming home, Sarah was once again climbing the apple tree in our backyard, and showing off her three tiny scars to anyone who wanted to look.

But on another level—and maybe I say this because as Sarah's dad, and a nonmedical professional, I felt this was the only part of the process that was my responsibility, that it was my job to be on top of—my daughter's appendectomy opened my eyes to the nightmare that is our nation's health-care system. Because when the bills and insurance statements started rolling in—a snow squall of papers featuring incomprehensible phrases like "patient encounter summary" and "allowed amount" and "core network" and "out-of-pocket cost"—I struggled to understand any of it. And this wasn't a case where coverage was being denied, or the doctor had left his BlackBerry inside my daughter's belly. No, this was a case where everything went *right*.

Which is why I set out to understand it—not just Sarah's bill, but why what I was being asked to pay for her care, what the insurer was paying, what we were paying *for*—was so hard to figure out. I discovered two things: first, that much of the cost of our health care is determined behind smoked glass, where patients are never invited to look. And second, that in trying to make sense of a single simple case where everything went right, you can learn a lot about what's wrong with health care in America.

ANY PHILADELPHIAN WHO'S been inside Children's Hospital will tell you it's an institution at once breathtaking and heartbreaking. On the breathtaking side, the only thing I can compare it to is Disney World, which—no matter where you stand on it philosophically—is without question the cleanest, friendliest, most competently run operation in the entire history of humankind. CHOP, I can say confidently, runs a close second.

As for the heartbreak? Well, it strikes you the minute you walk through CHOP's sparkling glass facade and start striding its sunny, brightly painted corridors. There are kids here who will spend years as patients in this place, and some of them will never go home. If there's a deeper level of hell than being the parent of a gravely ill child, I can't fathom what it might be.

Deirdra Young oversees billing and payment for all those patients. She's a soft-spoken middle-aged woman, and she works, not in CHOP's main building on 34th Street, but in space CHOP rents in the Wanamaker Building near City Hall, in an office adjacent to a sea of cubicles so large it's almost comical. I went to see Deirdra one day with a sheaf of papers under my arm and a simple plea: Help me, Deirdra, feel less like a dunce.

The first paperwork related to Sarah's surgery arrived a couple of weeks after she came home. Since the health coverage I get as a staffer at this magazine is what's known as a high-deductible/health savings account plan—that is, I'm responsible for the first $4,000 of annual costs, which I pay out of a health savings account to which I make monthly contributions—I braced myself, expecting to see a vast total cost of which, hopefully, I'd only have to pay a petite proportion. I saw neither. The paper, from my insurance company, United Healthcare, read:

Radiology Services $71.00

Network Discount $14.20
Amount Allowed $56.80

I was baffled at first, but then secretly gleeful, the way you feel when you're speeding and you pass a cop but for some reason he doesn't pull out and come after you. Could it be this was it—the only bill I was going to get? That somehow everything Sarah had gone through—the ultrasound, the surgery, the IVs, the three nights in the hospital—had slipped through the billing cracks? She was small. It was possible.

Over the next few weeks, unfortunately, I started seeing and hearing the lights and sirens that haunt a wanted man. Every day when I came home from work, a new bill or statement from my insurance company was waiting for me—most of them either indecipherable or contradictory. There was a bill for "anesthesia services" of $1,326, yet the amount due was only $1,060, though neither I nor my insurance company had paid anything so far. There was a bill for "radiology services" that seemed to indicate the $209 charge was covered by insurance, but another identical one that indicated it wasn't. My favorite showed up in December: It listed a charge for room and board of $3,100, then another for "IH miscellaneous services" of—drumroll, please—*$19,742.16*. I wondered whether my five-year-old daughter had been force-fed Kobe beef throughout her hospital stay, or maybe had been ordering up porn on pay-per-view.

Now, sitting with Deirdra Young, I dove into my stacks of paper and asked her to explain it all to me. I started with that bill for CHOP's radiology services of $71 that had been adjusted down to $56. Deirdra looked at it, then patiently explained what I now know to be the First Rule of the American Health-Care System: Insurance companies don't pay retail.

"Your insurance plan has some kind of contractual agreement with us, where we're going to adjust your charges by a certain amount," she explained. So United Healthcare gets its own set of prices—prices that don't have much to do with what's on the bill? An X-ray isn't $71, it's only $56? "Right. We have contracts with different payers. And the contract may say—I'm trying to make this as simple as possible—that for this procedure, we're going to give you a 10 percent or 20 percent discount. It varies by contract."

This little bit of information—which maybe you knew but I didn't—helped clear up the confusion on a number of Sarah's bills. Her anesthesia bill was $1,326, but thanks to the discount, we only owed $1,060. The surgery bill was $3,235, but the discount knocked it down to $2,059. The more bills Deirdra and I went over, the more I started to feel proud of my insurance company: *Look at you, United Healthcare, all gettin' me a deal and shit.*

I moved on to some of the statements I'd gotten from United that didn't seem to match up to any bills from CHOP. It was then that Deirdra taught me the Second Rule of the American Health-Care System: There are a ton of bills and charges that we, as consumers, never see. For instance, Sarah's Kobe beef bill—the $19,000 in miscellaneous services? Turns out I'd never gotten an actual bill from CHOP for that because United Healthcare was picking up the tab.

This made me feel pretty good, but out of curiosity, I asked Deirdra just exactly what those $19,000 in charges were *for.* She called up Sarah's account on her computer. "All of this," she said, turning the screen so I could see it. The charges were now broken down by 12 different "revenue codes." For instance:

Pharmacy—General $1,978.97
Emergency Room—General $554

And while to me these charges seemed monolithic, Deirdra further explained that there was an itemized breakdown for each one. A moment later, her screen filled with line after line of charges that looked like the federal budget. I asked her if she could print it all out for me. She raised her eyebrows. "You're not going to understand what these abbreviations are. You're fine with that?"

"I'm fine with that," I said. She handed over a printout, and I realized she was right. Most of the line items—95 in all—were gibberish. Thiopental, $53.25. Endo Stapl*, $547.19. Finally I saw one I thought I could understand: Hot Pack, $36.

For the first time in the entire process, I realized, I was seeing Sarah's actual bill. This was the full accounting of everything that had been done to my sweet little daughter.

What was truly fascinating, though, was that this list of charges was more or less useless. Of the $19,000 in miscellaneous charges, my insurance company had paid only $4,954. "It's the contract," Deirdra explained. In fact, while the total charges for Sarah's stay were $28,738, United and I only paid about $12,000 ($9,136 from United, $3,233 from me). Sixty percent of the charges vanished into thin air.

Figuring out just what an insurance company pays for and what it doesn't isn't cheap. Physicians for a National Health Program, a group pushing for national health insurance, says paperwork and bureaucracy account for nearly a third of every dollar we spend on health care—and that streamlining the system could save nearly $400 billion per year.

At CHOP, more than 60 people work for Deirdra Young in her department. She has them divided into different groups, each one working with a different insurer, since each insurer has its own peculiar codes and ways of doing things. "In this business, you have to have a good relationship with the payers," Deirdra said. "We meet with them every four to six weeks, and we have spreadsheets, and we look at what are the denials, is your system set up right, did something change."

I asked: Does she ever wonder if there's a better way to do all this? She laughed. "Some days I do say that—when I look at some of the issues we have. Can't we just keep it simple? But

I don't think we're there yet. It would be good if we had one system, one payer. I just don't think we're there."

I AM, IT seems, not the only Philadelphian or American flummoxed by the complexity of the health-care system. In fact, as medicine grows more sophisticated and complicated, we're quickly approaching a crisis point in what experts call "health literacy"—our ability to comprehend everything from the instructions our doctors give us to our insurance claim forms. "It relates not just to understanding the medical terms, but to the consumers' need to understand the system of health care and their responsibilities to pay for health care," Madeline Bell, CHOP's chief operating officer, told me one day on the phone. "So what you're experiencing is that it's a complex system, and you don't have a high level of health literacy—because it's not something that most people have. Even me. I feel I'm educated about it, but when I'm a consumer, I really have to take my time and understand all the components of it."

I called Madeline a couple of days after talking with Deirdra. I wanted to ask her two things: First, how did CHOP go about calculating what I'd started thinking of as the "sticker price"? Second, how did CHOP and United Healthcare figure out how much CHOP should actually get paid?

The sticker-price portion, it turns out, isn't particularly difficult to grasp. Madeline explained that CHOP looks at "acquisition costs"—that is, what it has to pay for things like drugs, supplies, workforce—then adds in data regarding what's typically charged for a service—in short, the going market rate. That seemed logical enough. What I found curious, though, was this: United Healthcare wasn't the only one who got a break on the cost. No one ever pays full price.

"That's not how it works," Madeline said, with a little bit of a laugh. "It sounds strange, I know. But it's typical that hospitals have charges, then they'll negotiate a contractual agreement with insurance companies. You won't get a situation where the insurance company will pay the charges. That's just how this system works."

Now, I'll admit to being a little bit of a wiseass here, but I couldn't help wondering—and apparently I, uh, did this out loud—just why the hell a hospital would establish a price that no one on the planet was actually going to pay.

"Well, it helps us understand what our gross revenue is," Madeline responded politely. "It's just a system that's been set across the board for health care. There are some systems"—she stopped, and it was clear that this was much more complicated than I was ever going to be able to understand. She explained, for instance, that sometimes what insurers paid was a percentage of the retail price, although sometimes it wasn't. . . . "I think it's just a long-standing system. I know it doesn't make sense to the general consumer."

Actually, it made perfect sense: The price is what it is because that's what the price always was—well, except when it isn't.

I moved on to my other big question: If sticker price is irrelevant, then how do hospitals and insurance companies figure out how much the insurers—and, by extension, all of us—actually pay? The answer turns out to be one that any mass-market merchandiser would understand: Typically, the more customers an insurance company has, the better the deal it gets from a health-care provider like CHOP. "For those insurance companies where we do a high volume of service, there will be more of a volume discount," Madeline explained.

That our health-care system operates on the same economic model as Sam's Club—with a family pack of appendectomies costing less per item than one solo appendectomy—was not particularly comforting. Indeed, it struck me as exactly the opposite of the way things should be. Doesn't giving price breaks encourage people to use the health-care system more? Madeline told me that in some areas of the country, hospitals are experimenting with variations on the current model. One is what's called "outcome-based payment"—where a hospital gets paid a better rate if everything goes the way it's supposed to, with no infections, say, or a patient gets out of the hospital after a set number of days. The other burgeoning trend is insurance companies not paying for what the industry ominously calls "never events"—that is, the hospital doesn't get paid if the patient dies when he or she wasn't supposed to.

Honestly, I have no idea what to think about that.

I liked Madeline Bell, and I could tell she is genuinely sympathetic to how complicated all of this is to the average patient. She explained, for example, that CHOP was as open as possible with families when it came to helping them get a grasp on costs. "We give families the information they need to understand their bill," she said. "The problem is, many times it creates more confusion." After looking at Sarah's 95 line items, I could understand that. That said, Madeline told me there are cases where delving into every one of the charges in detail is crucial: "There are some health plans out there that have lifetime maximums. And if you have a child who's chronically ill, it's important that you understand what your insurance company is paying for in your child's care."

GIVEN THE DIFFICULTY I was having understanding one simple, successful appendectomy, I can't imagine what it must be like for those families whose stays at CHOP are measured in months, not days, and whose bills climb into the hundreds of thousands of dollars and beyond.

And what happens if you have no insurance at all? Families that can afford to pay cash get a 20 percent discount. If you can't afford to pay anything, CHOP offers a variety of options, including a charity-care program. While a portion of every bill goes toward subsidizing those cases, Madeline said there was no way for her to say what the exact percentage was. (Philanthropy also helps cover the cost of charity care.)

"This is how things have evolved over time," Madeline said of the system in general. "Nothing will drastically change unless

we have a different person in office and blow up the entire system of health care and have universal health care. Then, things
will change."

In the meantime, CHOP is playing by the current rules. A
few minutes after I got off the phone with Madeline, a woman
from CHOP's public relations department called me and—in a
move that says everything you need to know about what a business health care is—told me there was some concern Madeline
might have said too much about how CHOP figures out its rates
with insurance companies. Please don't print how much the hospital gets paid for specific services, she implored. It could hurt
CHOP in its negotiations with other insurance companies.

GIVEN THE AMOUNT of health care Americans consume—in 2007,
we spent $2.3 trillion on it—I've come to realize that Sarah's
successful surgery wasn't the only miracle that happened last fall.
The simple fact that her bills were processed—and processed
without any denials or complications, other than the fact that I
thought my head was going to explode—was astonishing.

"We handle 300 million claims per year," said Daryl Richard,
a vice president at United Healthcare, when I called for some
insurance-industry perspective on both Sarah's bills and the
entire Gordian knot of a system.

One of the ways United avoids being overwhelmed by that
kind of volume is by removing human beings from the process
as much as it can. The charges Sarah rang up at CHOP, for
example, were sent electronically to United Healthcare, where
a computer determined whether the charges seemed valid and
signed off on how much to pay. Daryl told me that 82 percent
of the company's claims are "auto-adjudicated"—meaning no
person has to get involved. It's simply one computer talking to
another.

Given that, I asked how United knew that all of Sarah's
charges—all 95 line items, $29,000 worth—were legitimate. I
had no reason to suspect they weren't, and frankly, I wasn't going

to fight CHOP even if something was fishy, but I wondered how much of a leap of faith United is willing to take.

"One of the roles we play, for the employers and consumers we serve," he explained, "is to make sure we administer your benefits correctly—so that you're not overcharged, or undercharged, and that your plan is covering what should be covered.

"And I think you highlight such an important issue, because—and I'm quite impressed with how much you dug into this—because I wish there were more consumers who were taking the time to understand their benefits and claims. Health care is going to continue to be a fairly complex system. But part of the way we can simplify it is if our consumers become more educated about how these processes and systems work."

This "empowering the consumer" is something United is really big on. Daryl told me, for example, that the company's website has a calculator that tells you how much a particular service or procedure should cost in your particular area of the country. He also said that starting this year, the company has come up with new claims statements designed to be much simpler for patients and their families to understand.

THE NOTION THAT for our health-care system to work properly, we all need to be savvier consumers seemed to me exactly right ... and exactly wrong. Yes, half of what's whacked with our system is its mind-numbing complexity and lack of transparency, which not only add billions in costs but make it impossible for anyone to behave like a rational consumer. How can you know whether a drug is overpriced when it's so hard to find out the price in the first place?

And yet I certainly don't feel confident that smarter health-care choices would necessarily mean lower premiums. Last year, for instance, even as it bemoaned the rising costs it was paying on behalf of its members, United Healthcare's parent company made a profit of $4.1 billion.

Which leads to what may be the other fundamental flaw of our health-care system: the fact that we treat it as a capitalistic enterprise at all. Would it have made any difference if I had known the final cost of Sarah's appendectomy ahead of time? I suspect I speak on behalf of most of the parents who pass through CHOP's breathtaking, heartbreaking halls when I say: There is no amount of money I wouldn't pay to see my kid get better. If you had told me on the night of Sarah's surgery that I had to empty out my 401(k) to pay for it, I would have done it. Sell my house? Yup. Borrow thousands from friends and family? In a heartbeat. Buy a gun and knock over a liquor store? If that's what it took. Some things are more powerful than business, more powerful than money, more powerful, frankly, than right and wrong. And that may be precisely what makes our health-care crisis insolvable: We are trying to put a price on something that is, by its nature, priceless.

ONE RECENT FRIDAY afternoon, I sat down with Peter Mattei, the surgeon who took out Sarah's appendix. Peter is a 43-year-old Harvard Med School grad whose jet-black hair and dark eyes make him look like a central casting version of Surgeon. I caught him on his lunch break, after a morning in which he'd done five surgeries.

He seemed embarrassed to admit he knew little about the billing and payment part of his profession. He explained, for example, that he's a salaried employee of his surgical group, so whatever United Healthcare and I paid for Sarah's surgery certainly hadn't gone directly into his pocket.

We talked for a few minutes about his life as a pediatric surgeon—he does about 500 procedures a year, ranging from simple mole removal to treating kids with cancer—and then about the complexity of the system that brought us together one night last October. We agreed that there must be a better way to do this—though neither of us knew what that might be.

There was a time, long ago, when a surgeon like Peter Mattei would have operated on Sarah, then sent me a bill for what his services cost. I would have sent back a check, or worked out a way to pay what I could over time. It was a previous generation's way of resolving the contradiction between what is, on the one hand, a business and, on the other, a basic human need. People seem capable of doing that; complex bureaucracies, not so much.

I'd brought with me my folder of the paperwork on Sarah's case, and I started showing it to Peter. He noticed the itemized listing of charges—her real bill—and asked if he could take a look at it. He seemed fascinated by the list, finally zeroing in on some of the charges directly related to what had gone on in his operating room.

"Wow, an endostapler costs $550?" he said, referring to the device he'd used to close Sarah's wounds, that had left such tiny little scars. Then the man who'd saved my kid, a guy I could never repay no matter how much I paid him, shook his head in disbelief. "That's amazing."

Mind Bomb

Kevin Baker

From *New York Magazine*

If you had a fifty-fifty chance of carrying a mutant gene that causes a fatal brain disease, would you want to know?

SOMETIME ABOUT THIRTEEN years ago, my mother's brain began to shrink. The signs that something was wrong proliferated slowly, but as ominously as something out of a science-fiction movie.

My mother became unaccountably restless and unable to concentrate. She complained constantly that Larry, my stepfather, didn't take her out anywhere, that they never did anything—although she could no longer follow the conversation at a dinner party and said things that other people found incomprehensible. She tried going back to work in some of the little tourist shops where she lived, in Rockport, Massachusetts. My mother worked most of her adult life, but now she couldn't figure out how to run a cash register or follow the simplest directions. Each time, she was fired after a few days, returning home baffled and indignant.

She was becoming indignant a lot. She began to fly into a rage at the smallest frustrations, cursing at herself and at other people in words we never heard her use before. She started to drink as well, something else she had never done much before. My mother had been a classic half–a–glass–of–Champagne–on–New Year's Eve drinker. Now she had to have wine every night, and even a little made her garrulous and belligerent.

It was as if every part of her personality was being slowly stripped away, layer by layer. The loving, gentle woman my sisters and I had known was being replaced by someone we did not recognize.

There were other things going on as well, physical changes. Her speech was often slurred, even when she was not drinking. Her movements became jerky and exaggerated, as if she could no longer fully control her limbs. She could not abide any restraints. During a drive one Christmas afternoon, I watched while she sat in the passenger's seat, compulsively buckling and unbuckling her seat belt, again and again, for over an hour. She kept complaining about how it stuck against her body, as if she had never seen or used a seat belt before.

My youngest sister, Pam, and I persuaded her to see a doctor. Her primary-care physician thought she knew what was wrong and sent her to a neurologist to confirm it—but at the last minute my mother refused to keep the appointment. Instead she went on drinking and growing steadily more impatient with everything and everyone around her. She shoved a woman she thought was crowding her at an airport baggage carousel, swore at people over parking spaces.

Mostly she fought with Larry. When he tried to stop her from drinking, she became incensed, threatening to burn down the house they owned together or to blacken over the paintings he sold at a local gallery. Their fights became wild and vitupera-tive. She accused him of being the one with a problem, of being a depressive, of stifling her. A certain mania seemed to come over her during these arguments. Once she did a sort of Indian war dance around him, challenging him to fight.

"I told him, if you want to fight, my family knows how to fight!" she told me. "You ain't seen nothin' yet!"

Around that time, I went to Boston to try to intervene. I remember it was a beautiful spring day and we were walking around Beacon Hill. She seemed delighted to see me, but all I could notice was how strange she acted. She hadn't had a drink, but her gait was wobbly and her eyes looked glazed. She no longer seemed to understand how the stoplights worked. Repeatedly, I had to reach out and pull her back from walking straight into traffic. We strolled down into Boston Common, where a homeless guy on a bench made some innocuous passing comment to her. My mother, always the most private, the most dignified of people, stopped and twirled around, doing a little pirouette for the homeless man, beaming the whole time.

Soon afterward, Larry confronted her with an empty wine bottle she had secreted in their closet. She wrenched it from his hand and hit him across the face with it, cutting his nose. He needed stitches to close the wound, and while he didn't press charges, my mother had to appear in court under the domestic-abuse laws. I hired a defense lawyer, who got her off with a warning, and finally we prevailed on her to go to a neurologist. This was a full eight years after we first noticed dramatic changes in her behavior. The tests revealed what her primary-care doctor thought all along: My mother was suffering from Huntington's disease.

Huntington's (HD) is a hereditary disease, its most illustrious victim the folk- singer Woody Guthrie. It's caused by a defective gene that produces a mutant "huntingtin" protein. The protein is necessary to human development, but its mutant version produces an excess of glutamines, amino acids that begin to stress, then eventually kill the brain's neurons. Huntington's is also known as Huntington's chorea, or "dance," for the florid movements that are its most obvious symptom. But such movements do not afflict all sufferers, nor are they the illness's most destructive characteristic.

Huntington's is a "profound" disease, one of the few neurological disorders that attacks nearly every area of the brain, says Steven Hersch, an associate professor of neurology at Harvard Medical School and Massachusetts General Hospital, and my mother's neurologist. It affects the cerebral cortex, where thought, perception, and memory are stored. It also shrinks the basal ganglia, which serves as a sort of supercomputer for the rest of the brain, regulating almost everything from movement to the input and output of thoughts, feelings, emotions, behavior. The result is what Hersch terms a loss of "modulation" and "a coarsening" of how we do just about everything—move, think, react. Huntington's sufferers have trouble correctly reading emotions in others or even recognizing familiar faces. They no longer understand when their behavior is inappropriate, and have difficulty planning, organizing, and prioritizing. They can become both intensely angry and apathetic and indecisive.

"They're losing possibilities," says Hersch. "They're losing the possibilities of things they could do, or think of, or want to do."

Not the least of Huntington's effects is what the knowledge of the disease does to its victims. There is no cure. Adult- onset Huntington's usually afflicts individuals sometime between 35 and 55, although early-onset, or juvenile, Huntington's can manifest itself before the age of 20. The disease commonly takes ten to thirty years to run its course, as body and mind slowly shut down and leave the sufferer all but inert. Before that happens, victims commonly die from major infections, pneumonia, choking, or "silent pneumonia," as food goes down the wrong pipe.

Suicides are not uncommon, even among "at-risk" patients who have yet to actually ascertain that they have the disease. Depression is also frequent among such individuals. If one is faced with such a fate, denial can be a survival strategy.

"Often the people who do best are those who can wall it off and go on with their lives," acknowledges Hersch. "It's a very good approach in a lot of ways. The trick for people sometimes is to figure out when it's in their best interest to drop the denial and gain knowledge that will help them."

The test results devastated my mother. Before long she reverted to denial. She insisted that her test had produced "a false positive." She told us that she had "the syndrome of the disease, but not the disease itself." She told us that, somehow, she was "the control" in the test. But as her brain continued to shrink, she began to lose even these words. It became a little joke between us.

"Dearest, I don't have this, you know," she would tell me, very seriously, out of the blue. "I'm the—the . . ."

"The control?"

"Yes, that's it!" she would say, delighted.

"Mom, you can't be the control if you can't remember the word *control*," I would tell her, and she would laugh, and I would laugh. But a few minutes later she would tell me again that she didn't really have this, you know.

The fact that my mother had Huntington's meant that I had a fifty-fifty chance of inheriting the gene—and thus the disease—myself. I didn't like to look at this too directly. That was my own form of denial. I told friends and relatives that I would not take the genetic test that my mother had taken. What was the point, without a cure? It could only screw up my health insurance, and who wanted to live with such a fate hanging over their head?

But those 50-50 odds worked their own havoc. Eventually I found that I couldn't help thinking about the disease whenever I had trouble coming up with a word or organizing an article. I noticed whenever my body flinched involuntarily. I became especially aware of how often I would drag one of my feet along the sidewalk, or how frequently my left arm would twitch. I took to holding my left hand out in front of me, trying to reassure myself by seeing how long I could keep it still—a better test for delirium tremens, I suppose, than Huntington's disease.

"Would you stop doing that? You don't have it!" Ellen, my wife, would tell me.

Yet I was sure that I could feel something deep inside me, something that I came to think of, a little melodramatically, as a stirring. Sometimes, lying awake in bed late at night, I was sure that I was only holding it back by force of will. I was certain that if I let go, I would begin to move compulsively, uncontrollably, just as my mother did now. The dance.

"I think I might have this," I told Ellen.

"I don't think you do," she said.

But her assurance was based on wishful thinking, or the sort of baseless conception one often has about someone else's life. My wife didn't want me to have the disease, and she thought of me as a lucky person, somebody who just wouldn't get such a thing. Yet none of this mattered. In reality, unlike fiction, people's lives don't run according to some overarching narrative. We never suspected this disease was in my family before my mother was tested, we didn't think of ourselves as shadowed by some sort of gloomy, gothic fate. But nonetheless, here it was.

I kept surreptitiously doing my little tests. Should I forget me, may my left hand lose its cunning. . . .

Every step of the way, meanwhile, my mother's denial only made everything worse for her. It now meant the dissolution of the life she had made with Larry—the quiet days in retirement they loved to spend fishing or reading and watching the news together in the evening; going to their favorite bakery every Sunday morning. None of it was enough to appease what was going on inside her brain. She wouldn't stop sneaking drinks, wouldn't keep taking the medications the doctors prescribed to control her moods. We would have been happy to let her drink if that had helped her, but the alcohol only stressed the brain and served to dilute the effects of the drugs. My mother now demanded almost constant attention to keep her entertained, to keep her from wandering into disaster. Eventually Larry told us he wanted out. They had been married for 21 years, and my mother had nursed him through a heart attack, cancer, and occasional bouts of epilepsy. But Larry, an émigré from Middle Europe, had seen both the Nazis and the Communists march into his life, and he knew when to head for cover. I couldn't blame him. It's an enormous burden for any one person to take care of a Huntington's victim, particularly someone who is a senior citizen himself, and he had been dealing with it for a decade. Pam and I hired more lawyers to negotiate the divorce, the sale of their neat little house, the overwhelming thicket of bureaucracy that determined where and how she might live now.

Pam managed to find her a nice studio apartment in an assisted-living facility in Beverly, Massachusetts; a converted high school with the pretentious name of "Landmark at Oceanview." (Just what was the "landmark"? The last leg of the voyage before you ease into the good harbor of death?) There were big school windows that brought in lots of light, and bright, cheery carpeting, and a diligent staff to make sure that she took her pills and to cook her meals and do her laundry—all tasks that she was having increasing difficulty performing.

Personally, I wanted to shoot myself every time I set foot inside the place. My mother, on the other hand, thought it was unbelievably "posh," the sort of home where she had always dreamed of living.

Meanwhile, my father, whom she had divorced nearly 30 years ago, came east with cinematic notions of getting remarried and taking care of her. He disregarded almost everything we told him about Huntington's and instructed her that she should just try to concentrate on holding her limbs still. Before one ghastly family dinner in a restaurant, he let her have a drink, then tried to cut her off. When his back was turned for a moment, she calmly snatched up his full wineglass and downed the contents in one swallow. I saw his eyes widen. My mother spent the rest

of the meal barely able to speak, rolling her head back to try to
get food down, until we made her stop out of fear she would
choke to death in front of our eyes. My father fled back to his
apartment in Hollywood. Good-bye, Golden Pond.

I was determined by this time to face the disease head-on. If
my mother had made everything worse for herself by remaining
in denial, I would throw it off. I would take whatever medications
were necessary, volunteer for whatever experimental programs
there must surely be. I convinced myself that this was a purely
practical idea. Why go about looking for cures or ways to ameliorate the effects of the disease if I didn't have the gene? Looking
back now, I think my decision may have been more emotional
than anything else, a desire to know this and be done with the
uncertainty. I told myself I would be stronger than my mom, and
take whatever I was given. Early in 2007, I set up an appointment
at Columbia University's HDSA Center for Excellence, located
up in Washington Heights.

The Columbia Center deals with every aspect of the disease,
both for those already suffering from HD and for those at risk,
and it endeavors to help patients through each stage. It's unique
in that the care it offers is free, although there are nominal fees
for some parts of the gene test. The center's testing protocol,
established and refined over the fifteen years since the Huntington's gene was first identified, is actually an involved process,
one that takes place over a few months—and is an infinitely
better one than what my mother went through. One of its chief
purposes was to slow me down—to let me think over what I was
doing. As the center's genetic counselor warned me at the start,
"Once you know, you can't not know."

There was the session with the genetic counselor, a visit to
a psychiatrist, neurological and neuropsychological exams. If
after all that I still wanted to know, they would draw my blood
and tell me the result of the gene test. That result would be a
number—the number of times a particular string of glutamine
DNA, known as CAG, repeated itself at the beginning of my

Huntington's gene. If that number was 27 or below, I was in the clear. If it was 36–39, I would fall into a tiny percentage of the population that might, or might not, develop the disease. If it was 40 or more, it meant that I had inherited the defective gene—and that I would get the disease.

I threw myself eagerly into the testing process, glad now to be doing this, to be confronting these phantom fears. The not knowing by now had become as bad as knowing the worst could possibly be, I told myself. I disavowed everything I had told people before. Best to look this fate in the eye, to see if it really was waiting for me.

The initial exams went well. The doctor found no signs that I had the disease already (my twitching left arm promptly stopped twitching so much). But the doctor seemed less than pleased that I was taking the test at all. The genetic counselor had insisted that there was no right or wrong reason for wanting to take the gene test, but it seemed clear that I had made the wrong choice.

Later, I found that I had misinterpreted the doctor's attitude. There really was no right or wrong reason to get the test, she was simply a little surprised by my motives. Most of the people they saw came because of some life trigger. They were making career decisions, getting married, thinking of having children—or wanting to spare their children, now marriage age, from having to take the test. Or they had just learned that Huntington's was in the family, or that a genetic test existed.

Getting tested so that you could see what you could do about the disease was unusual . . . in part because there is currently nothing you can do to cure the disease or even curb its progress.

Huntington's is what the federal Food and Drug Administration (FDA) officially calls an "orphan disease"—it affects too few people to make it worth the drug companies' while to develop a drug for it on their own. The official cutoff number is 200,000 people; Huntington's currently afflicts only 30,000 to 35,000 people in the United States, with perhaps another 200,000 to 250,000 at risk of getting the disease.

The National Institutes of Health (NIH) provide subsidies in such cases, but the total amount spent in the U.S. on finding a cure this year will probably be no more than $120 million to $130 million. A substantial sum, to be sure—but not so much when you consider that it can easily cost drug companies $1 billion to come up with an effective drug. As it stands now, a cure is not on the horizon. The most promising idea seems to be "turning off" the defective Huntington's gene, but discovering how to do that presents a host of technical problems that remain far from solved.

The doctor's surprise at my motives drew me up a little short—not a bad thing. Getting tested for the gene of a hereditary disease with no cure is and should be a hugely complicated decision, one with implications beyond one's own self. It can mean "outing" other family members, who may have no desire to learn if they will get the disease. It can mean any number of problems with one's health insurance (no doubt a big reason why fewer than 3 percent of at-risk Americans get tested for HD, as opposed to 20 percent of Canadians who might have the gene). It can mean dealing with unanticipated feelings of guilt, dread, despair. It all made me think again. Was I engaging in a reckless act of bravado, moving into a realm that I was not psychologically or emotionally prepared for, just to show that I could do it?

"No matter what the result is," my genetic counselor warned me, "nobody is the same person they were when they walked in here."

I was pretty sure that if the results were negative I would be the same person I was in about five minutes. On the other hand, the 50-50 chance that I had the gene had already begun to unravel any peace of mind about my future. Bravado or not, I had to know. I had them draw the blood. They told me it would take two to four weeks for a result, depending on how crowded the lab was. No matter what the verdict was, I would have to come back to the clinic for the counselor to tell me in person.

During my trips to the Columbia Center, Ellen and I would sit in the plain, institutional waiting room and watch other outpatients coming and going. Some displayed no outward signs of having the disease; others clearly had the telltale movements. Some of these people carried themselves with remarkable bravery, others were so young that it was almost unbearable to watch them. I knew that, in a very short time, I would either walk away and never see them, never see this place again, or that I would join their small fraternity.

The two to four weeks that I had to wait seemed to stretch out like a lifetime—in the best sense of the words. I put the possibility of having the gene out of my head again, and was more sanguine about my chances than I had been in months, still buoyed by the revelation that all my twitching had been, so to speak, in my head.

Only one afternoon, while I was working in a library, did the full understanding of what I was doing sneak up on me. What if it really is positive? I thought to myself, out of the blue, and I realized that I had no answer. I was stepping over a cliff, into a state of mind that I had no real way of even imagining. I quickly went back to my research, shutting this idea safely away again behind my own walls. But it was still there.

When the call came two weeks later to set up my appointment, I wished for more time. I had two days to wait. I joked with my wife that our appointment was on an auspicious day—the anniversary of Hitler's invading Russia. But I also couldn't help wondering, "If it's negative, wouldn't they tell you over the phone? I mean, even if they say they won't? Just to give you peace of mind, as soon as they can?"

"No, they have a whole procedure," my wife insisted. "It's going to be fine, you don't have this."

"But I'm just saying. Wouldn't you tell the person? Wouldn't it be sadistic to let you wonder for the next two days if the news was good?"

"It's a procedure!"

We took the subway up to the center and got there a little early, seating ourselves in the waiting room again. Almost as soon as we arrived, my genetic counselor came out to see us-and we had our answer. When she walked into the waiting room we could both see that tears were welling up in her eyes, and that her mouth was set in a tight little smile, like someone trying to pretend there's nothing wrong. It was like being on trial and having a jury come back that won't look you in the face. After that, it was all over very quickly. The counselor sat us down in her windowless office and told us at once that the number of my CAG repetitions was 41—one number higher than my mother's. I had the defective gene, and my brain, too, would begin to die.

I can't say that I was immediately stricken or horrified. I didn't even feel as upset as I have sometimes when an editor hasn't liked a manuscript. It felt, as bad news often does, as if I'd known what it was going to be all along. Outside, it was still a sunny early-summer day. We got back on the subway. Ellen tried to be consoling, but I wasn't in need of any, not just then. What was there to say? When we got home, I got a call from a podiatrist wanting to move up an appointment for a minor foot problem I was having. I hustled over to the East Side and there I sat, in another doctor's waiting room, not an hour later. It all seemed unreal, like some weird simulation of what I had just been through. I thought about how giddy I would have been feeling if the results had been negative. I felt like blurting out the news to anyone I encountered, *I just found out I will get a fatal disease.* But I didn't. The doctor prescribed some egg cups for my shoes, and I went home.

A couple days later, the bottom fell out. I was working at my desk when I began to doubt every single thing that I was writing. I was certain that I was already losing my ability to think, to put together a simple sentence. Later that night, lying in bed, I was gripped by a terrible, souring sense of dread, a feeling that everything in my life was useless, meaningless. I had never experienced anything like it before. I am a person of faith and optimism, at least when it comes to my personal outlook, but all that gave way before this wrenching, physical sensation of despair. This feeling came over me several more times during the week after my test. Nothing, not even the most soothing and optimistic thoughts I mustered, could ameliorate it. I wondered if this was what true, clinical depression felt like.

Then it would fade away and I would feel strangely exhilarated, just as one does when a fever passes. I learned to ride these moods out, just try to get through them, and soon they largely disappeared. I was, I suppose, building a new wall. All that brave confrontation, just to escape behind a new layer of denial! Nonetheless, everything did seem more intense, more edged. My moods were more mercurial, I was angrier, more sympathetic, even more apathetic about things—always aware that these very mood swings, too, were symptoms of Huntington's.

I made predictable resolutions. I would live more in the moment. I would hone my life to the essentials; read more great books; stop wasting so much time on newspapers, the latest catastrophe from Africa or China, or the op-ed pages. Who had time for it? Instead, I would write and write and write, build a legacy of work.

Yet this soon created its own sense of panic. I had easily twenty, thirty, maybe more good ideas for novels, histories, screenplays—how would I ever get all that done? What I really wanted was to live like I always did, taking little care of myself, wasting time worrying over politics, or how the Yanks were doing, or even the banality of other people's opinions. As a novelist I learned long ago to pace myself, building something day by day, rewarding myself along the way with all the sweet distractions of modern, urban life. I wanted my trivialities. I kept thinking of the title of that self-help book, something like *Don't Sweat the Small Stuff—and It's All Small Stuff.* But of course it's the small stuff that we crave. That's what gives us the illusion that life is infinite, the only thing that saves us from the terror of consciousness, the root of which is that uniquely human knowledge that we are going to die. My mother's denial did indeed make everything worse for her, and at times it tormented those of us who loved her. But now I found her stubbornness, her desire to cling to the life she had known, understandable, even admirable.

I started to tell people about my test results, what they meant. This made my wife uncomfortable, but I couldn't help myself. I had some kind of compulsion to tell friends, family, even professional acquaintances. I wasn't sure why I felt this need. Was I trying to solicit their pity, their admiration? *See how brave he's being!*

Probably. But I think I was also doing it out of sheer incredulity, or even as a cry for help. *Here I am dying. Do something!*

My friends duly praised my courage—as if I had any choice. They spoke about all the great things going on in medicine today. I nodded and smiled, told them yes, I would pursue every cure. But there are no cures, at least not yet, and I doubt that a nation bent on spending three or four trillion dollars on the grand task of making the Iraqi people learn to love one another is ever going to devote much more to solving my little brain ailment. For that matter, I can't honestly say that my disease should have any priority over the likes of breast cancer, strokes, heart disease, or any number of other maladies that affect many more people.

All things considered, I knew that I had already had a phenomenally good life. Even when it came to the Huntington's, I had been lucky enough not to live with the disease hanging over my head. I was never somebody who worried about death or thought about it much at all. My wife and I had fortunately decided not to have children, a decision we reached more or less by inertia over the years and which meant that, thank

God, I didn't have to worry about having passed this on to someone else.

And yet, inevitably, I would find myself filled with rage at times. I thought maybe it was the knowing that made all the difference. I joked about the old Woody Allen lines, from *Love and Death*: "How I got into this predicament I'll never know . . . To be executed for a crime I never committed. Of course, isn't all mankind in the same boat? Isn't all mankind ultimately executed for a crime it never committed? The difference is that all men go eventually. But I go at six o'clock tomorrow morning."

But I wasn't going tomorrow morning. No one is sure what triggers the onset of Huntington's. The gene's interaction with other genes, or environmental factors, or even aging itself may play a role. Heredity and especially gender seem to be very strong factors. The disease could begin to take its toll at almost any time, but because I inherited it from my mother instead of my father, it is more likely to manifest itself around the same age when she got it, at 65 or maybe even older—a very late onset.

"The brain copes, until it can't anymore" is the exquisite phrase with which Herminia Diana Rosas, an assistant professor of neurology at Mass General and Harvard Medical School, describes the progress of the disease. Huntington's may well be active in the brain ten, even twenty years before any symptoms begin to show up. We don't see its effects because the brain rallies to adjust. In a touchingly human response to this threat, the neurons compensate by trying to do less, or by sharing vital information among each other, squirreling away knowledge and memory where they can.

In other words, I had not received some fatal diagnosis, not really. All my Huntington's gene guaranteed was that I was going to start to die, most likely at the same age that many people start to die, from one thing or another, prostate or heart disease, stroke or diabetes or Alzheimer's—much as we are all dying, all the time. I might have another good sixteen years ahead of me, maybe even more. I joked that it was like being on death row, only with better company. I joked that it was like being on death row, only with better food. Coming out of my agent's building on yet another gorgeous summer day—and what a beautiful summer it was—I told myself, "You'll be doing this ten years from now, and you'll still have six years to go. Think of how long that is, how much will happen and how much you can do!"

What I really feared was not death but what would precede it. Dr. Hersch's "coarseness" meant a lack of nuance—a great prescription for a writer. I would be unable to work, to organize my thoughts or comprehend the world around me. I would forget friends, names, faces, facts, memories. I would be unable to control my moods, my movements, my urges, would become a living caricature of my former self—much like what I had seen happen to my mother.

Our efforts to get her to adjust to life at her assisted-living facility were breaking down. She became belligerent if she felt she was being mistreated or thwarted in any way. She kept insisting that she wanted to be married again, kept pursuing men of any age. When someone told her that a 95-year-old fellow resident at Landmark had said she was nice, she harassed him to the point where she had to be forcibly removed from his room, slugging a female staff member in the process.

This time she was ejected from the facility. After a brief and volatile stay in a nearby nursing home, my mother was shipped out to a psychiatric ward, where she was drugged nearly to the point of being insensible. She couldn't speak, could barely move, and seemed to be experiencing hallucinations. My sister, noticing other inmates walking around dressed in some of her clothes, raised hell, cajoled doctors, and managed to get her transferred to a much better facility, a sprawling state hospital. It was a place with light and space and a dedicated staff that adjusted her medication so that she was alert and talking again. She seemed much happier, the violent rages ebbing away, but all the transfers, and the progress of her disease, had taken its toll. She had trouble completing even a simple sentence, and her gait was so unsteady that she was confined permanently to a wheelchair.

There was no disguising that she was in an institution now. Her ward was all tile and linoleum, and she was surrounded by other inmates suffering from advanced neurological disorders, Huntington's and Parkinson's, multiple sclerosis, retardation, and dementia. There was one man, younger looking than my mother, who just sat about with his head crooked permanently to one side, his tongue lolling out of his mouth. Another woman, all but immobile, told us how she had been a nurse for many years but was now suffering from Parkinson's. She seemed to be alert enough and in her right mind.

Which was better? To be past any awareness of your condition—or to be sinking slowly into it, still conscious? I wondered what the point was of trying to extend the longevity of the human body before we knew more about preserving the mind. How much would I understand when I was put in some institution like this? Ellen swore that she would take care of me at home, and I knew she meant it. But I also knew that in the end, she would not be able to do so, that this was my fate I saw here before me.

Visiting my mother was an ordeal to me now. And yet it also felt oddly soothing to just sit with her in silence, while she patted my arm and smiled at me, saying little. It occurred to me that she was tracing the path I would follow. It reminded me of *The Vanishing,* that creepy European film in which a man is so guilt-stricken over not knowing what became of his lover that he allows her psychotic killer to kill him in the same extended, horrifying manner, just so he can know what she experienced. When my mother first went to live at Landmark, my sister persuaded her to give up her car; her deteriorating physical skills made her a menace to herself and to others on the road. But Pam gave her a few weeks first to get used to the idea, to ease her transition to living on her own, in a strange town, at the age of 75. My mother would usually drive back to Rockport, a place she loved, a place where she had lived for nearly 40 years, and where she no longer belonged. There she would just sit in her car, out on the town wharf, and watch the gulls circling and diving over the harbor. I often thought of her there, and now I understood that I would, one day, know what she was going through.

A Huntington's drug trial materialized late last year at a Mass General clinic up in Charlestown, Massachusetts—the first interventionary test ever, for at-risk subjects who as yet had displayed no symptoms of the disease. I volunteered immediately. The trial consisted mostly of taking daily supplements of creatine, the bodybuilding drug, which, it was thought, might strengthen and extend the life of neurons. It wouldn't "cure" the disease, but at my age, preserving as many brain cells as possible—buying time—might prove almost as beneficial.

The first step was another battery of tests, starting with an MRI. When it was over, I got to see a picture of my brain for the first time. Dr. Rosas, who runs the program with Dr. Hersch, her husband, told me that there were no visible signs of Huntington's yet and pointed out the caudate nuclei, the parts of my brain that were most likely to shrink first. They lay along the edges of the pool of cerebral-spinal fluid that separates the left and right hemispheres of the brain—an area that looks like a pair of dark wings on the MRI, delicate and beautiful. I stared at them for a long time, thinking of how someday the wings would lose their shape as my brain shrunk and they expanded, leaving only more of the blackness.

There was something else on the scan as well. A little white circle, maybe half the size of a dime. Dr. Rosas wanted to know if I'd had any headaches or violent seizures recently. I had not, but it seemed the suspicious little dot could be a tumor in the making. More tests would be required, through my primary-care physician back down in New York. Oh, and it also seemed that I had a cataract in each eye.

I left the clinic in Charlestown before they could diagnose me with malaria or dengue hemorrhagic fever. It took most of a month to get a more detailed cat scan and learn the results. I didn't really think I had a brain tumor, since I didn't have any symptoms. I told myself, half-joking, I *cannot* get two brain diseases in the same year. But I knew enough now not to try to outguess the tests, and the waiting began to drag on me. A few days into the New Year, I went to get those cataracts looked at. They proved to be no real problem, so small now there was nothing to be done but wait for them to grow. Still, coming back from my ophthalmologist's, I could barely see through my dilated pupils; struggling to dial the number on my cell phone for the MRI results that were due back that same day. Staggering blindly up Riverside Drive, on a blustery January day, the wind whipping at my face and hair, I had to laugh, thinking how my life was turning into a road production of *King Lear*.

This time, the news was good. I didn't have a brain tumor. The little white dot was nothing at all. One brain disease to a customer. There was life, there was hope. There was the recognition that all I was going through—the torment of an aging parent, the knowledge that I would likely follow in her footsteps—was really nothing that unusual in our America of aging seniors and genetic testing. What was to be done but to make the most of it?

Back at home, I looked at the scan with my wife. "I'm going to miss that brain," she said.

"I know," I told her. "I'm going to miss me, too."

The Uneven Playing Field

Michael Sokolove

From the *New York Times Magazine*

BY THE TIME Janelle Pierson sprinted onto the field for the start of the Florida high-school soccer playoffs in January, she had competed in hundreds of games since joining her first team at 5. She played soccer year-round—often for two teams at a time when the seasons of her school and club teams overlapped. Like many American children deeply involved in sports, Janelle, a high-school senior, had traveled like a professional athlete since her early teens, routinely flying to out-of-state tournaments. She had given up other sports long ago, quitting basketball and tennis by age 10. There was no time for any of that, and as she put it: "Even if you wanted to keep playing other sports, people would question you. They'd be, like, 'Why do you want to do that?' "

Janelle was one of the best players on a very good high-school team, the Lady Raiders of St. Thomas Aquinas High School in Fort Lauderdale. A midfielder and a 2007 first-team, all-Broward-County selection, she had both a sophistication and a fury to her game—she could adroitly put a pass right on the foot of a teammate to set up a goal, and a moment later risk a bone-jarring collision by leaping into the air to head a contested ball.

That she was playing at all on this day, though, was a testament not to her talent but rather to her high threshold for pain, fierce independence and formidable powers of persuasion. Janelle returned to action a little more than five months after having an operation to repair a ruptured anterior cruciate ligament, or A.C.L., in her right knee. And just 20 months before that, she suffered the same injury to her other knee.

The A.C.L. is a small, rubber-band-like fiber, no bigger than a little finger, that attaches to the femur in the upper leg and the tibia in the lower leg and stabilizes the knee. When it ruptures, the reconstructive surgery is complicated and the rehabilitation painful and long. It usually takes six to nine months to return to competition, even for professional athletes. But after her second A.C.L. operation, Janelle refused to wait that long. When her teammates were at practice, she felt a longing. What were they doing? Who was playing well? What jokes were they cracking? Just about every girl pictured in her hundreds of photographs from homecoming and other social events was a soccer team-mate. She missed her sport, her friends, her life. Whenever she started to feel depressed, she said, "I would just try to rehab harder and get back earlier."

Janelle's mother broached the subject with her of whether she should continue playing at all. "I'm afraid for her, and for all these girls," Maria Pierson told me recently. "What's it going to be like for them at 40 years old? They're in so much pain now. Knees and backs and hips, and they just keep going. They've been going at this so hard for 10, 11, 12 years, and it's taking a toll. Are they going to look back and regret it?"

Janelle's father was concerned, too, but a bit more philosophical. Title IX, the federal law enacted in 1972 mandating equal opportunity in sports, has helped to shape a couple of generations of girls who believe they are as capable and as tough as any boy. With a mix of resignation and pride, Rich Pierson said to me: "We've raised these girls to be headstrong and independent. That's Janelle."

Janelle told her parents that she was still determined to play soccer in college—and that she would race through her rehab in order to salvage the end of her senior season in high school. Her physical therapist thought that was a bad idea. Her surgeon was reluctant to write a letter to her school stating that she was medically cleared to resume playing, but Janelle persuaded him.

Playing through pain, rushing back from injury—a warrior-girl ethos—was ingrained in Janelle, just as it is in many young women. The more she was hurt, the more routine the injuries felt. Her first A.C.L. operation, she told me, was "monumental. It felt scary. You know, it's surgery." Then she added: "The second one was like, O.K., I know what I need to do, let's just do it. Let's have the surgery and rehab and get back out there."

By Janelle's and her mother's count, her club team, with 18 players, had suffered eight A.C.L. tears—eight—during her high-school years: Janelle's two, another player's two and four other girls with one each. A high-school teammate one class above Janelle endured chronic ankle problems and, according to a Miami Herald article, six ankle operations—three in each leg—over the course of her four years on the varsity soccer team.

This casualty rate was not due to some random spike in South Florida. It is part of a national trend in the wake of Title IX and the explosion of sports participation among girls and young women. From travel teams up through some of the signature programs in women's college sports, women are suffering injuries that take them off the field for weeks or seasons at a time, or sometimes forever.

Girls and boys diverge in their physical abilities as they enter puberty and move through adolescence. Higher levels of testosterone allow boys to add muscle and, even without much effort on their part, get stronger. In turn, they become less flexible. Girls, as their estrogen levels increase, tend to add fat rather than muscle. They must train rigorously to get significantly stronger. The influence of estrogen makes girls' ligaments lax, and they outperform boys in tests of overall body flexibility—a performance advantage in many sports, but also an injury risk when not accompanied by sufficient muscle to keep joints in stable, safe positions. Girls tend to run differently than boys—in a less-flexed, more-upright posture—which may put them at greater risk when changing directions and landing from jumps. Because of their wider hips, they are more likely to be knock-kneed—yet another suspected risk factor.

This divergence between the sexes occurs just at the moment when we increasingly ask more of young athletes, especially if they show talent: play longer, play harder, play faster, play for higher stakes. And we ask this of boys and girls equally—unmindful of physical differences. The pressure to concentrate on a "best" sport before even entering middle school—and to play it year-round—is bad for all kids. They wear down the same muscle groups day after day. They have no time to rejuvenate, let alone get stronger. By playing constantly, they multiply their risks and simply give themselves too many opportunities to get hurt.

Janelle's first-round playoff game in January took place at Lockhart Stadium in Fort Lauderdale; the temperature was in the mid-70s, and there was a light breeze, the kind of weather that inspires people to move to Florida. Janelle, with a bulky black brace on her right knee, dressed for the game against the better judgment of her parents. "They were like, 'No, you're not going to do that,' " she said. "And I was like: 'Yes I am. This is my last year, and I want to win the state championship.' "

Her knee was still a little stiff, she said, but she put that in the category of "aches and pains." She told me after the game: "You have to learn to deal with pain, because if you don't, you'll never get to play. It's not like you ever feel perfect."

Janelle began the game on the bench because her coach, Carlos Giron, promised her parents to limit her playing time to no more than 25 or 30 minutes of the 80-minute match. She was not in the kind of overall shape to play a whole game, and besides, the contest was not expected to be much of a struggle. Under Giron, the Lady Raiders had already won 10 state titles. But the game started out tighter than expected, and 15 minutes into a scoreless match, he motioned for Janelle. As she came bounding off the bench, her mother, next to me watching from the bleachers, audibly exhaled.

Maria Pierson, the owner of a public-relations firm, loved watching Janelle play over the years and was never bothered much when her daughter was knocked to the ground or even bloodied in collisions. Now, though, she was a total wreck. "Oh, God, I have such a stomachache," she said. "I can't stand it." When Janelle and an opposing player went for a ball at midfield and it looked as if they would arrive at the same moment, her mother emitted a high-pitched yelp, then uttered something like a prayer: "Please don't kick her in the leg. Please."

A few minutes later, Janelle collided with an opponent. Her right knee, the one most recently surgically repaired, was extended out in front of her body as she tried to get her foot on the ball. This finally sent Maria Pierson over the edge.

"No! No! Oh, no!" she yelled. She jumped up from her seat and her sunglasses went flying off her head into the row below. Janelle emerged unscathed. Her mother retrieved her glasses and exhaled. For the moment, Janelle was fine.

PARENTS OF TEENAGE girls who play sports have grown accustomed to what seems like entire teams battling injuries—and seeing those who do make it onto the field wrapped in Ace bandages or wearing braces on various body parts. Hannah Cooper, a star soccer player at Bethesda-Chevy Chase High School in Maryland, sat out several games early in the 2007 season with a severe ankle sprain, one of many she has suffered since her years in middle school. "The left one never fully recovers, so I play in a brace," she told me not long ago. "I also have shinsplints, so that hurts all the time, but I've just learned to ignore it. I also tore my meniscus, or I think I did," she said, referring to knee cartilage. "I've probably had concussions because I've had hard collisions where I was disoriented and had headaches afterward, but I've never missed a whole game because of one. If I have to sit out, I always come back in."

David Cooper, Hannah's father, observed: "I once heard that the injury rate in the N.F.L. is 100 percent. It looks to me, in girls' soccer, it's the same thing."

On a night soon after Hannah returned to action last fall against crosstown rival Walt Whitman High School, two of her teammates sat out because of their own ankle sprains. But that was nothing compared with the injuries on the Whitman team, which competed without five key players—two were finished for the season with ruptured A.C.L.'s, two were sidelined with concussions, and one was out with an injured back.

Whitman's senior captain, Rachel Haas, did play, and was her team's most visible player because of her remarkable, almost freakish throw-ins. Whenever her team was deep in its attacking end, Rachel was able to fling the ball all the way into the goal area—a potent offensive tactic made possible by the extreme flexibility of her spine. When she took the ball back behind her head to throw, and arched her back, she looked like one of those old Gumby dolls you can bend in any direction. Rachel's mother said her daughter regularly visited a chiropractor, and that chronic back pain had cut short each of her previous three school seasons.

Rebecca Demorest, a sports-medicine pediatrician, told me that it is common for her to treat young women with injuries from head to toe. "They ache and they hurt and they use pain medicine and try to keep on playing," she said. "When they finally get to the point they can't play, they come in to see me. . . . They have a series of nonspecific, overuse injuries that comes down to being worn out. Don't get me wrong. There's a chain of events with boys too. But I see it more with the girls." (I spoke with Demorest when she was based at Children's Hospital in Washington; she has since moved to the Women's Sports Medicine Center at the Hospital for Special Surgery in New York.)

Comprehensive statistics on total sports injuries are in short supply. The N.C.A.A. compiles the best numbers, but even these are based on just a sampling of colleges and universities. For younger athletes, the numbers are less specific and less reliable. Some studies have measured sports injuries by emergency-room visits, which usually follow traumatic events like broken bones. A.C.L. and other soft-tissue injuries often do not lead to an E.R. visit; the initial examination typically occurs at the office of a pediatrician or an orthopedic surgeon. Studies of U.S. high-school athletics indicate that, when it comes to raw numbers, boys suffer more sports injuries. But the picture is complicated by football and the fact that boys still represent a greater percentage of high-school athletes.

Girls are more likely to suffer chronic knee pain as well as shinsplints and stress fractures. Some research indicates that they are more prone to ankle sprains, as well as hip and back pain. And for all the justifiable attention paid to concussions among football players, females appear to be more prone to them in sports that the sexes play in common. A study last year by researchers at Ohio State University and Nationwide Children's Hospital in Columbus, Ohio, reported that high-school girls who play basketball suffer concussions at three times the rate of boys, and that the rate for high-school girls who play soccer is about 1.5 times the rate for boys. According to the N.C.A.A. statistics, women who play soccer suffer concussions at nearly identical rates as male football players. (The research indicates that it takes less force to cause a concussion in girls and young women, perhaps because they have smaller heads and weaker necks.)

But among all the sports injuries that afflict girls and young women, A.C.L. tears, for understandable reasons, get the most attention. No other common orthopedic injury is as debilitating and disruptive in the short term—or as likely to involve serious long-term consequences. And no other injury strikes women at such markedly higher rates or terrifies them as much. Rachel Young, a former soccer player at Virginia Tech who had to stop playing after two A.C.L. ruptures and substantial cartilage damage in her right knee, told me that young women she knew feared the injury but rarely talked about it. "A.C.L. is like a curse word," she said. "You just cringe when you hear it."

An A.C.L. does not tear so much as it explodes, often during routine athletic maneuvers—landings from jumps, decelerations from sprints—that look innocuous until the athlete crumples to the ground. After the A.C.L. pulls off the femur, it turns into a viscous liquid. The ligament cannot be repaired; it has to be replaced with a graft, which the surgeon usually forms by taking a slice of the patellar tendon below the kneecap or from a hamstring tendon. One reason for the long rehabilitation is that the procedure is really two operations—one at the site of the injury and the other at the donor site, where the tendon is cut.

Janelle suffered her first A.C.L. injury at practice with her club during a routine drill. When she planted her left leg to shoot, the knee buckled. Her mechanics felt no different than they had thousands of times before: Decelerate. Fix on the target. Kick. There were few things in her life she did with more ease or joy. Her second A.C.L. injury occurred the following summer at the annual Texas Shootout in Houston, a prestigious event that attracted 300 teams and 360 college coaches as well as major corporate sponsorship, including Adidas, Gatorade and the Texas Sports Medicine Center. In the first game, she ruptured the A.C.L. in her other knee. "This time I was pretty sure what it was," she said. "I was chasing after this girl, trying to cut to stop her. And it just went out on me."

She stayed down on the field, screaming. A trainer came out and tried to calm her, assuring her the pain would subside. But her screams came more from anger than pain. She instantly understood that most of her senior season of high-school soccer would be wiped out and worried that no college coach would want to recruit her. (What she did not realize was that if college coaches shunned girls with a history of serious knee injuries, they would struggle to put quality teams together.)

The nature of both her A.C.L. injuries—occurring, as they did, without contact and seemingly in the absence of any extraordinary circumstances—is the very thing that perplexes A.C.L. researchers. It takes 2,000 Newtons (a measure of force) to rip an A.C.L. apart. (Researchers know this from intentionally snapping cadaver knees.) The mystery is why a knee works properly for many years—through game after game, practice after practice, long season after long season, for tens of thousands of repetitions—and then, without warning, a tiny but crucial component suddenly malfunctions.

Steve Marshall, a professor at the University of North Carolina's School of Public Health, leads a large A.C.L. study financed by the National Institutes of Health that is following students at the three major U.S. military academies. The idea is to take a series of measurements—as well as to study digitized images of a student's form when landing from jumps—and then to build an "injury group" from among those who go on to tear their A.C.L.'s. What traits did they have in common? And which of those traits can be modified so that the rates of injuries can be lessened?

"I'm an injury epidemiologist, and I've been doing this for a while now," Marshall says. "This is the first time I've studied something where I can't show you what did the damage. If we were reconstructing an incident where a child fell down a staircase, I could say, 'O.K., he got a laceration here because of where he hit the handrail.' Or he rolled his ankle, or whatever. If it's a car crash, you say, 'O.K., the road was slick, a crash occurred and a loose object in the car came up and hit someone on the head.'

"But here, you can look at a video of an injury all day long, and what you see is people in the air. People landing. People cutting. What we can't actually see is what tears the thing apart."

If girls and young women ruptured their A.C.L.'s at just twice the rate of boys and young men, it would be notable. Three times the rate would be astounding. But some researchers believe that in sports that both sexes play, and with similar rules—soccer, basketball, volleyball—female athletes rupture their A.C.L.'s at rates as high as five times that of males.

Anthony Beutler, a major in the U.S. Air Force and a professor at the School of Medicine of the Uniformed Services University in Bethesda, Md., is among the cadre of doctors, scientists and researchers trying to crack the code of A.C.L. injuries. In 2001-2, he was a sports-medicine fellow at the Naval Academy, where he served as the physician for the women's soccer team. Seven women were lost that season to A.C.L. ruptures. Beutler, already immersed in A.C.L. research, was still stunned. "I thought to myself, What in the heck is going on here?" he said. Last season, the women's team at Navy suffered three torn A.C.L.'s. "They thought that was great, a fortunate year," he told me. "Think about that. Just three. It's bizarre."

Men also tear their A.C.L.'s, most frequently in football and from direct blows to the leg. But even football players, according to N.C.A.A. statistics, do not rupture their A.C.L.'s during their fall seasons at the rates of women in soccer, basketball and gymnastics. The N.C.A.A.'s Injury Surveillance System tracks injuries suffered by athletes at its member schools, calculating the frequency of certain injuries by the number of occurrences per 1,000 "athletic exposures"—practices and games. The rate for women's soccer is 0.25 per 1,000, or 1 in 4,000, compared with 0.10 for male soccer players. The rate for women's basketball is 0.24, more than three times the rate of 0.07 for the men. The A.C.L. injury rate for girls may be higher—perhaps much higher—than it is for college-age women because of a spike that seems to occur as girls hit puberty.

If you are the parent of an athletic girl and live in a community that bustles with girls playing sports—especially the so-called jumping and cutting sports like soccer, basketball, volleyball and lacrosse—it may seem that every couple of weeks you see or hear about some unfortunate young woman hobbling off the field and into the operating room. The first time, you think: What a stroke of bad luck. But you figure it won't happen to your daughter because, after all, what are the odds?

After a couple of more A.C.L. tears in the neighborhood, you get worried and think, Gosh, we must be in a really bad cluster for these injuries. Why here? But in all likelihood, what you are witnessing is not a freakish run of misfortune but the law of averages playing out.

The Injury Surveillance reports include commentary as well as data, and in 2007 the authors stated that an A.C.L. rupture is "a rare event" and advised against making too much of the tears sustained by male and female collegiate athletes across a range of sports. But a young woman playing college soccer can easily generate 200 exposures a year between her regular season in the fall, off-season training in the spring and club play in the summer. Plenty of younger players, girls in their early through late teens, will accrue well in excess of that number between their high-school seasons, their club seasons—which often run year-round—and multigame tournaments on weekends and soccer camps in the summer. (The same is true in other sports in which girls play school and club seasons, including basketball, lacrosse, volleyball and field hockey.)

So imagine a hypothetical high-school soccer team of 20 girls, a fairly typical roster size, and multiply it by the conservative estimate of 200 exposures a season. The result is 4,000 exposures. In a cohort of 20 soccer-playing girls, the statistics predict that 1 each year will experience an A.C.L. injury and go through reconstructive surgery, rehabilitation and the loss of a season—an eternity for a high schooler. Over the course of four years, 4 out of the 20 girls on that team will rupture an A.C.L.

Each of them will likely experience "a grief reaction," says Dr. Jo Hannafin, orthopedic director of the Women's Sports Medicine Center at the Hospital for Special Surgery in New York. "They've lost their sport and they've lost the kinship of their friends, which is almost as bad as not being able to play."

Marshall says he feels a sense of urgency, because without a better understanding of the injury, the situation will get worse in coming years with the great numbers of girls playing sports—and the frequency and intensity of their play. In 1972, at the dawn of Title IX, about 300,000 girls participated in high-school sports. The number is now three million. Thirty thousand women played college sports pre-Title IX; about 205,000 now play.

"We're studying an elite population at the service academies, but the big concern for me is the girl down the street who wants to play soccer on the rec team or the travel team," Marshall told me. "They're ripping their knees up, and they shouldn't be. There's got to be a way to prevent it. And we're really on the up curve of this, because it's still relatively recent that girls played sports in these large numbers. . . . So if you think we have a problem now, 10 years from now we'll have a much bigger problem."

ONE WEEKEND IN the Fall of 2007, I watched a soccer match involving two teams of 13-year-old girls in Southern California with Holly Silvers, a physical therapist and the director of research at the Santa Monica Orthopaedic and Sports Medicine Research Foundation. These were elite players, but from one end of the field to the other, Silvers pointed out girls she judged to have insufficient core muscle strength, balance or overall coordination to play safely. Their movement patterns put their knees—and probably their ankles, hips and backs—at risk.

"Look at the girl on the left back with the ponytail," she said as we stood on the sideline of a game at the Home Depot Center, a vast complex of fields in Carson, Calif., where the men's and women's national soccer teams train. "She really concerns me." At first I couldn't pick out whom she meant; there were lots of ponytails out there. "No. 8," she clarified, and I fixed my attention on a tall, stiff-legged girl whose upper and lower bodies seemed not to be in communication with each other. She ran bolt upright, with very little bend in her trunk. Her knees seemed not to flex. When she came to a stop or slowed to change directions, she landed flat-footed. "She's got really poor form," Silvers said. "She won't hold up running like that."

She pointed out another girl with possibly even worse form. She was one of the better players on the field, but Silvers said her advanced skills masked serious physical flaws. I asked her if she could fix the girl, given the opportunity. "Yes, I could," she said. "In four to six weeks I could improve her a lot. In three months, I could get the job done. I would educate the muscles, educate the nerves. She could build strength and change her patterns."

Silvers directed my attention to one more player, a girl who seemed light on her feet, quick and springy. When she changed directions, she stayed in what generations of gym teachers have called "the athletic position"—knees bent, butt low to the ground. Even when walking casually during stoppages in play, she seemed more lithe than the other girls. "She moves more like a boy," Silvers said. "Believe me, that's a good thing."

Silvers, along with a Santa Monica orthopedic surgeon, Bert Mandelbaum, designed an A.C.L.-injury-prevention program that has been instituted and studied in the vast Coast Soccer League, a youth program in Southern California. Teams in a control group did their usual warm-ups before practices and games, usually light running and some stretching, if that. The others were enrolled in the foundation's "PEP program," a customized warm-up of stretching, strengthening and balancing exercises. An entire team can complete its 19 exercises—

including side-to-side shuttle runs, backward runs and walking lunges—in 20 minutes. One goal is to strengthen abdominal muscles, which help set the whole body in protective athletic positions, and to improve balance through a series of plyometric exercises—forward, backward and lateral hops over a cone. Girls are instructed to "land softly," or "like a spring."

There is nothing complicated about the program. And nothing really exciting about it either—which, as with many preventive routines, is one of its challenges. As essential as it may be, it's not as interesting as kicking a soccer ball around.

The Santa Monica Orthopaedic and Sports Medicine Research Foundation published results of its trial in the American Journal of Sports Medicine. The research was nonrandomized and therefore not the highest order of scientific research. (The coaches of teams doing the exercises made a choice to participate; the control group consisted of those who declined.) Nevertheless, the results were attention-grabbing.

The subjects were all between 14 and 18. In the 2000 soccer season, researchers calculated 37,476 athletic exposures for the PEP-trained players and 68,580 for the control group. Two girls in the trained group suffered A.C.L. ruptures that season, a rate of 0.05 per 1,000 exposures. Thirty-two girls in the control group suffered the injury—a rate of 0.47. (That was almost twice the rate for women playing N.C.A.A. soccer.) The foundation compiled numbers in the same league the following season and came up with similar results—a 74 percent reduction in A.C.L. tears among girls doing the PEP exercises.

The program has direct parallels with the research taking place at the military academies. Both are focused on biomechanics—the way athletes move—in no small part because gait patterns can be modified, unlike anatomical characteristics like wider hips. Marshall has been encouraged by information taken from the sensors attached to his subjects as they jump. "Women tend to be more erect and upright when they land, and they land harder," he said. "They bend less through the knees and hips and the rest of their bodies, and they don't absorb the impact of the landing in the same way that males do. I don't want to sound horrible about it, but we can make a woman athlete run and jump more like a man."

Silvers stressed the importance of training girls as young as possible, by their early teens or even younger. "Once something is learned neurally, it is never unlearned," she said. "It never leaves you. That's mostly good. It's why motor skills are retained even after serious injuries. But ways of moving are also ingrained, which makes retraining more difficult with the older athletes. The younger girls are more like blank slates. They're easier to work with."

The PEP program, and others like it around the country, are not without their skeptics, who ask how you can try to solve a problem before you are even confident of its cause. Donald Shelbourne, an Indianapolis orthopedic surgeon and researcher, is perhaps the most vehement of the critics. "It's like me taking antioxidants," he says. "I don't have cancer yet, so it's working, right? These retraining programs play on emotions without data. They're unproven. Jumping and landing is something that everyone knows how to do, and now we've got people saying, 'We can teach you to do it better.' I don't buy it."

Coaches rarely like to give up precious practice time for injury prevention, and often have to be pushed by parents. As Diane Watanabe, an athletic trainer who is part of the Santa Monica research team, puts it: "Coaches have to see a performance boost. Otherwise, they won't do it. That's the only way we can sell them on this program."

The bigger barrier, though, may be political. Advocates for women's sports have had to keep a laser focus on one thing: making sure they have equal access to high-school and college sports. It's hard to fight for equal rights while also broadcasting alarm about injuries that might suggest women are too delicate to play certain games or to play them at a high level of intensity. There are parallels in the workplace, where sex differences can easily be perceived as weakness. A woman must have maternity leave. She may ask for a quiet room to nurse her baby or pump breast milk and is the one more likely to press for on-site child care. In high-powered settings like law firms, she may be less likely, over time, to be willing to work 80 hours a week. She does not always conform to the model of the default employee: a man.

Mary Jo Kane, director of the Tucker Center for Research on Girls and Women in Sport at the University of Minnesota, voices that sort of concern. "I'm not in any way suggesting that this topic should not be taken seriously," she says. "We need to do everything we can do to prevent injuries. But when you look at the stories that get told, that those who cover women's sports are interested in telling . . . it does seem that so little coverage focuses on women's accomplishments, on their mental toughness and physical courage. There is a disproportionate emphasis on things that are problematic or that are presented as signs of women's biological difference or inferiority."

Sandra Shultz, an A.C.L. researcher who teaches graduate courses in athletic training and sports medicine at the University of North Carolina at Greensboro, said she was more willing to focus on sex difference. "It depends on what side of the fence you're on," she told me recently. "If your job is to encourage inclusion of more women in sport, maybe you are not going to accentuate the negative. You don't want to paint women in a negative light and tell a girl that if you play sports, your knees, by the time you are 30 or 35, may be in bad shape. But intuitively, people know it. As a researcher and a clinician, I'm willing to talk about these things so we can do something about them."

Shultz and other researchers say that A.C.L. research and the training programs spawned by it may end up protecting women from a range of injuries—all of them stemming from poor form and underdeveloped muscle. "Just because a kid is good at a sport does not mean she has the foundational strength or movement patterns to stand up to constant play," she says. "What I'd like to be able to say is: 'Before you engage in a sport,

I am going to teach you how to move. And I am going to give you strength.' "

JANELLE, WHO TURNED 18 last month, told me that her teachers would consider her quiet but that she's a chatterbox with her friends. She is pretty, but not fussy about her appearance. She rolls out of bed in the morning, brushes her teeth, pulls up her hair and goes off to school. "Ten minutes," she says. "That's all I need. That's from the time I get up until I'm in the car."

She has a teenager's sardonic wit, and sometimes even her mother is not sure when she's serious. She went to a private Christian school when she was younger and now attends a Catholic high school. After taking a comparative-religion class this year, she told her mother that she might consider becoming a Buddhist, which Maria Pierson took as sort of a joke. "No, I meant it," Janelle told me. "I've been Catholic all my life. I don't know if it's the best religion. I told her I might go shopping for a new one, and I'm still actually planning on doing that."

Rich and Maria Pierson never had to push Janelle into soccer or to reach for higher-level teams, and they certainly never berated her after bad games. These types do exist, stereotypical "Little League parents," but it is far more difficult than some imagine to push a reluctant child into sports, especially at a level that demands great commitment. Children may acquiesce for a while, but all but the most passive or abused will eventually rebel and shut down.

I found a different syndrome: parents of highly motivated, athletic children who are supportive of their kids' sports but bewildered by the culture. The children, often as not, are the ones leading the way, and the whole family gets pulled along in ways it never anticipated. "We had no idea what we were getting into," Rich Pierson said. "You just feel your way as you go. She started playing with a local team, just once or twice a week, then began with the travel team, and after that it just builds on up."

Rich, a self-employed investor, told me his own childhood revolved around his parents' country club. The kids splashed in the pool, learned to golf, played baseball. "For my generation, this is the new country club," he said, referring to his deep involvement in youth sports. "It's where all your leisure time goes. It becomes your social set." (The Piersons have one other child, a son, now in college, who was also an athlete.)

In many sports, a youth athlete's paramount relationship is now with a club rather than a school team. Annual fees and travel to tournaments often run into the thousands of dollars. Parents pay for camps and private sports tutors. The guiding principle is that childhood sport is too important to be left to volunteers and amateurs. The quality of coaching, in terms of skills and tactics, is probably better than in past generations, but it is also narrower. Rather than being coached by educators who see them during the school day and have some holistic sense of them as children, young athletes are now mentored by coaches who cultivate only their athletic side.

At what age should a young athlete begin traveling to out-of-town tournaments? How many days a week should she be playing? When should she give up her other sports? The professional coach is usually not equipped to know what's best, but he wields tremendous influence all the same, sometimes by threat. He makes the schedules and sets the rules, and a child who does not go along risks losing her place on the team.

"Parents' hearts are usually in the right place," says Colleen Hacker, a sports-psychology consultant who has worked with athletes from the preadolescent up through the college, Olympic and professional ranks. "I don't think anybody's saying, 'Honey, how do we screw them up tomorrow?' But the attention, judgment and objectivity that parents bring to their work lives and other spheres of importance, they don't bring to their kids' sports."

The club structure is the driving force behind the trend toward early specialization in one sport—and, by extension, a primary cause of injuries. To play multiple sports is, in the best sense, childlike. It's fun. You move on from one good thing to the next. But to specialize conveys a seriousness of purpose. It seems to be leading somewhere—even if, in fact, the real destination is burnout or injury.

Anson Dorrance, the women's soccer coach at the University of North Carolina, is a fierce critic of the tournament system, which he says began when the women's game was young and good teams had to travel to find strong competition. "But now," he told me, "everybody's got a tournament. There's the Raleigh Shootout, the Surf Cup in Southern California, and ding, ding, ding, they're everywhere." Dorrance was animated, his words coming out in a rush. "So now girls are going somewhere every two or three months and playing these inordinate number of matches. And you know what? They're playing to survive. And the survival is not just the five games in three days. It's the two or three weeks following. They've got a niggling this and niggling that—sprained ankles, swollen knees, aching backs. They were overplayed and they never rested. But part of what's developing is this question of who's tough enough, who can play through it?"

Janelle suffered her second A.C.L. rupture, the one in Houston, while playing in her third tournament in three weekends with her club team, the Weston Fury. Each was a multigame tournament. The demands of a schedule like that—a dozen or more hotly contested matches over the course of three weeks (in three different states)—are beyond what is ever asked of any professional or collegiate team.

In Houston, she was among several players on her team still trying to attract the attention of college coaches. "There was maybe a little sense of panic," Rich Pierson says. "They were on the move, trying to be seen."

His daughter's injuries have caused him to reassess the intensity of youth sports. "There are worse problems, but this catches you completely by surprise," he says. "You don't see it coming. There's accountability all the way down the line. The coaches. The parents."

Janelle's high school, St. Thomas Aquinas, is the alma mater of the tennis immortal Chris Evert and the former football star Michael Irvin. It places a high value on attracting and developing young athletes, and on keeping them healthy enough to go on and play in college. "I get more compliance from the boys," the school's athletic trainer, Dwayne Owens, told me. "Boys are actually willing to sit if that's what I tell them. The girls want to get back out there. They want me to tape them up and let them play." I repeatedly heard similar sentiments from doctors, coaches and others: Girls are more likely to put themselves at risk. If they've played through a lot of pain in the past, they may be inured to it.

There is a fascinating parallel in research on injury rates in U.S. Army basic training, a two-month regimen that pushes recruits to their physical limits. In numerous studies going back more than two decades, women are shown to suffer injuries at substantially higher rates than men, with stress fractures to the lower legs a particular problem. But one large study also suggests that the women are both more frequently injured and tougher. It takes a bigger injury to knock them out of the service. The men, by comparison, are wimps; they leave with more minor ailments.

In sports, just as in the military, women are relative newcomers. In both venues, there may be an element of "toughing it out" to prove they belong. "From the earliest levels in girls' sports, up through the elite and Olympic level, how one plays the sport, how one comports oneself, is talked about in specific ways that transcend technical or tactical expertise," Colleen Hacker says. "It is more overt with the girls than the boys. Character counts. Physical toughness, mental toughness and handling adversity count."

When I was with Janelle, I could not help thinking of Amy Steadman, who was going to be one of the great American soccer players of her generation. In her junior year in high school, in Brevard, N.C., Parade magazine named her the top high-school-age defensive player in America, "the best of the best." She was a captain of the U.S. women's under-19 team, a future star of the women's national team. She played for Anson Dorrance at U.N.C., and while I was talking to him one day, he pointed out beyond his office door to a gallery where the uniforms of his all-time greats, including Mia Hamm, were displayed. "She would have been one of those jerseys out there," he said, referring to Amy.

But by the time I met her, Amy was 21 and had torn the A.C.L. in her right knee four times. The first time was when she was training for the under-19 World Cup. "That was my ultimate goal at the time," she told me. "I just wanted it so bad. I had 10 months to recover and get back to close to 100 percent, or I wasn't going to make the team. . . . I worked out like three or four hours a day. I was really determined, and being so young, I didn't know anything about patience."

Amy said that she had "a lot of complications" with the first one. But what she described in her understated way sounded more like a nightmare than complications. She briefly became addicted to her pain pills. She lost weight and became so dehydrated she had to be hospitalized and hooked up to an IV. She received a "huge lecture" from the nurses on how to take better care of herself.

But she achieved her goal and made the under-19 team, the highlight of her too-brief career. As Amy walked toward me the first time we met, her right leg was stiff and her whole gait crooked. She moved like a much older woman. If I hadn't known her history, I would never have believed she had been an athlete, let alone an elite one. She had undergone, by her count, five operations on her right knee. Her mother counted eight, and believed that Amy did not put certain minor cuttings in the category of actual operations. She was done playing. She had been told she would need a knee replacement, maybe by the time she turned 30.

Amy told me about her final operation, recalling that when she came out of anesthesia, the surgeon seemed as if he was going to cry. He looked at her in silence for what seemed like a long time, trying to compose himself. Finally, he told her, "Amy, there was nothing in there left to fix."

Janelle made it through that first playoff game, a 2-1 victory. But I sensed I was watching a shell of the player she had been and, with continued health, might be again. She was like an adult on the field—a supersmart, clever-passing, organizing presence—but she had no speed or explosiveness. Twice she passed up scoring chances because she would not plant on her surgically repaired knee to shoot with her left foot.

The next game, another victory, was on the Gulf Coast, but Janelle barely played. She did all that work to make it back so she could help her team in her senior year, but the game was fast and rough, and her coach went with younger players. On the long ride home across Alligator Alley, Janelle sat with a teammate in the back of her parents' S.U.V. but said hardly a word.

Later I asked if having so little playing time bothered her. "Yeah, of course," she said. "But those girls have been together for like 25 games without me. It's hard to break back into the lineup, and I have to try to understand that." I pointed out that she had been a first-team, all-Broward-County selection. "That was last year," she said.

Janelle played much more the next game, but the Lady Raiders lost—two games short of the state championship. Other girls cried. Janelle stoically walked off the field, unstrapped her knee brace and accepted hugs from her parents.

The next week, she began training at a privately owned gym. She had never before had anything that she construed as A.C.L.-injury-prevention training—and this was not labeled as such—but now she was working on her core muscles and doing exercises to improve her balance and her form when landing from jumps. From among the several colleges that vigorously recruited her, she settled on Lafayette, an academically select, Division 1 school in Easton, Pa.

In February, she competed again with her club team in the Score at the Shore College Showcase tournament in Tampa, an event that turned out to be a macabre example of the warrior-girl ethic—and a bizarre illustration of how youth sport exists within its own closed universe. On the first night of that tournament, a player on a team that had traveled down from Queens was struck and killed by a car as she crossed a busy highway to a convenience store for a snack. A teammate walking with her was hospitalized in serious condition. Their team decided to stay at the tournament and compete. The players wrote the dead girl's name on the sleeves of their jerseys and gathered in prayer on the field before the next game, which they won. The game goes on, no matter what.

In the semifinals, though, the Queens girls were shut out by the Weston Fury, Janelle's team. Janelle and her teammates were too emotionally drained to celebrate. Both teams just stayed on the field and cried. "It was horrible," Janelle said. "It was crazy. I don't even know why we were playing."

A couple of weeks later, Janelle suffered another injury—to her left knee, the site of her first A.C.L. rupture. She stepped awkwardly during a game, thought she heard something crack and felt a sense of panic. "I thought, I cannot believe I did this again," she said. An M.R.I. revealed a less dire diagnosis: she had "nicked" her cartilage, which would heal on its own after she rested for a few weeks. Her 18th birthday was coming up, and she felt as if she had just received an early present.

After three weeks' rest, Janelle planned to resume her physical training and not compete again until her college's first game late in the summer. But then again, her club team was entered in the State Cup in Florida. If the Weston Fury won enough games, it might still be playing into late May. Janelle figured she would be fully recovered by then. "If I felt like I could help my team," she said, "I might try to play."

That was still Janelle's mind-set: Rehab hard. Get back on the field. Compete fiercely. And hope not to be injured.

Blinded: What the Eye Doctor Didn't See

Grace Taulsan, J94, lecturer in English

from *Tufts Alumni Magazine*

THE WORLD I grew up in was riddled with dangers: snowballs, lollipops, drinking straws, metal clothes hangers, baseballs, tree branches, long-stem roses, popsicles, high-heel shoes, and the hardcover editions of books. Life was full of opportunities for blindness. My father saved up stories from his ophthalmology practice and transformed them into directives: Never rub your eyes. Always wear protective goggles. The threat here was "foreign bodies," which, despite his explanations, I pictured as miniature men in ethnic costumes kicking as he plucked them from the whites of his patients' eyes. And there were other rules: Don't allow the dog to lick your face. Never let a parrot sit on your shoulder, I don't care how well you think you know him. No jumping on the bed—look what happened to your brother.

Jon was almost two when he hit his eye on the corner of the wooden headboard and fell to the floor. It's taken decades for me to learn the details: how my father carried Jon through the emergency room of the hospital where he worked, past the waiting room and nurses' station. He set my screaming brother on a bed and pulled the yellow curtain around them. My father didn't trust the resident on call; apparently didn't trust anyone but himself to hold the pointy syringe, the threaded needle, and surgical scissors against the ripped skin under Jon's eyebrow.

My mother helped hold my brother down. My father sobbed as he sewed the stitches, but his hand was steady and careful. He understood how important the face is to human interactions, how a scarred and disfigured eye could jeopardize his son's future. The pink scar drawn underneath Jon's left eyebrow is a faded testament to my father's expert hands.

Now, 25 years later, I find myself pressed against the picture window on the seventh floor of Massachusetts Eye and Ear Infirmary. The Charles River shimmers, and for a weekday morning, a surprising number of sailboats glide in figure eights. It's a beautiful day in mid-August, a bittersweet day when we remember that summer will soon be gone.

Ten adults crowd this hospital room, missing meetings and not returning phone calls or emails so that we can sit around this empty bed. We're waiting for my two-year-old niece Joli to return from surgery to remove her right eye. The doctors are certain: it's cancer. Retinoblastoma.

My mother sits in a plastic chair, counting the hours in rosaries. In the spiritual equivalent of slipping cash to the hostess of an exclusive restaurant, she begs her dead parents and siblings to whisper in God's ear. Joli's other grandparents, the preacher and his wife, pray softly, and an occasional "praise God" or "in Jesus' name" rises to my ears. Joli's mother, my sister Liza, reads the latest Harry Potter, and Joli's father, Jorge, talks on the phone, telling and retelling the story for the hours we wait. We fear all the unknowns: how will Joli cope with only one eye? If they find cancer in both eyes, will she be blind? Has the cancer metastasized?

My brother Jon has just flown in from Maui. My other brother, Paul, a first-year medical student at Boston University, is skipping classes to sit with us. Alonso, my boyfriend of a decade, waits here, too. My sister Mari, who is due to give birth any week now, calls us constantly from Los Angeles for updates.

There's one puzzling no-show: my father, the ophthalmologist. We act as if his absence proves the depth of his love. My father must love Joli more than any of us does, and that's why he's not here.

But I know the truth. My father isn't here because he blames himself. If Joli dies because he waited too long before voicing his suspicions about the subtle, almost imperceptible changes to her eye that he alone among us could have interpreted . . . if Joli dies because my father didn't say a word and the cancer spreads . . . I will blame him, too.

On the morning Joli was diagnosed, it took only seconds. The pediatric ophthalmologist just blinked into his ophthalmoscope before announcing his suspicion: retinoblastoma. It's one of the few cancers that can be diagnosed upon visual examination. And just as quickly, my father, who was there chatting up his former colleague, spun around and left the room without saying a word. My father is the kind of man who can't let anyone know he cries.

My father didn't speak much for the rest of the day, nor did he leave the car to attend the flurry of appointments with specialists before my niece's operation the next morning. I was alone with him when he said miserably, "We could lose her."

"Not lose her," I countered. "Just her eye. That's the worst-case scenario."

"Losing her eye," my father said, "is the least of our worries."

My father stared at his hands as he told me a story. While in training for his ophthalmology specialty more than 30 years ago at Philippine General Hospital, he had witnessed enough cases of retinoblastoma to fear it. Some of the parents he met had read the mysterious white glow from their toddlers' eyes as a sign of special powers, an ability to divine the future or bring the family luck. "How stupid," my father said. By the time the sick children arrived from their remote provinces to Manila, it was too late, and they soon died. In 1975, when my father arrived in the United States to study at the Tufts–New England Medical Center (now called Tufts Medical Center), he immersed himself in science and distanced himself from folklore.

Once Joli was diagnosed, Liza recalled seeing a strange reflection in her daughter's right eye. Like the glow of a cat's eye. But the conditions had to be just right, and Liza didn't see it all the time, so it didn't alarm her. When we looked back over the many photos of Joli, we noticed a handful from the previous four months that showed hints of the white spot in her eye—photos my father undoubtedly never saw. The spot is there while Joli blows out two birthday candles. It's a little bigger while she's sitting with my father watching television after a summer cookout. We'd been taking photos of the cancer for months.

In the photo from the night before the surgery to remove Joli's eye, the tumor is plain as day. There is Joli, clutching a stuffed Tigger toy, her pupils still dilated from the exam. Where the flash should have produced the normal red-eye reflection, it has revealed something else. An opaque pearl, startling, beautiful, and deadly.

I didn't know how much I needed Joli until she was a year old. That's when she, Liza, and Jorge moved from New York to Boston, where I live. One day a week since then, Joli has been mine. I don't have children of my own, and it's fun to pretend. I leave my apartment before 7 A.M. so I can be the first to greet Joli when she awakes. I'm the one who performs the morning rituals of diaper change and warm milk bottle and snuggling. My name was one of her first words, and her parents taught her to add the Filipino word for aunt, Tita. As her vocabulary grew, I was Tee Grace, then Tee Tah Grace. And now she sings my name in a birdcall like the northern bobwhite, Tee Ta Grace.

My days with Joli have been some of the best of my life. We threw an entire box of cereal, a handful at a time, onto the living room floor and let her dog Gordie, the 170-pound Presa Canario, clean it up. We made snow by emptying a container of baby powder in her bedroom. We tossed pizza dough into the air and cracked eggs against the counter and spooned soil with ice cream scoops into seedling trays on the coffee table. After our day together, I feed and bathe her. I rock her on my belly and tell her a story, then continue retelling it, until Joli stops saying, Again, again, again.

Now, with Joli's diagnosis, I feel robbed. I want to say to my father, "You taught me to be afraid of pens and lollipops and snowballs and rosebushes and every sharp, pointed object in the world when all this time, the danger was inside of us, in the very cells of the eye itself."

When we tell the story of Joli's cancer to new people, my father is the hero. It was he who first noticed that Joli's right eye was slightly misaligned. During Easter holidays, I heard murmurs about strabismus, or lazy eye, and a month later my father began to share his suspicions regularly to any of us who would listen. At a Mother's Day meal, my cousin Rod, who is also a physician, admitted that he thought Joli was going cross-eyed.

Despite all the talk, no one was alarmed. We didn't want to consider that her misaligned eyes could threaten anything but her looks. Yet I wonder if silent alarms were firing in my father's head—Misaligned eyes! These could be symptoms of a rare eye cancer! My oldest sister was married that Memorial Day weekend, and all through the festivities, I noticed my father placing one hand, then the other, in front of Joli's eyes in what looked like a kind of game. Joli would swat his hand away in annoyance. "Leave her alone," I said. "She doesn't like that."

After Joli's diagnosis, my father, in a story he couldn't stop telling, insisted that he was doing that annoying hand trick to check Joli's visual field. "But she saw my hand," he said. "She saw it."

I understood what he needed. Forgiveness. Relief from culpability. "You couldn't have known," I said. And it's true. Only an eye exam with an ophthalmoscope would have caught the gooey tumors early as they started to gather and grow. Still, I wish he had said, "I doubt it's anything serious, but I've noticed Joli's right eye is wandering to the side. It's my professional recommendation that you take her to a doctor." After all, he routinely refers his patients to other eye experts when he understands his limitations as a general eye doctor. "I have to send you to Boston," he'll say. "They can take care of you there."

But with family members, fear and denial can get in the way. Perhaps he couldn't process what he was seeing: the loosening of Joli's focus as her eye drifted to the left. Perhaps he told himself it wasn't possible that his granddaughter's eye could fill with tumors, that her life could be threatened at the age of two. Who can blame him for wanting to deny his worst fear?

The irony is that my father, even though he is a doctor, doesn't believe in going to the doctor. His medicine cabinet is full of prescriptions he's written himself: antibiotics for sore throats and topical creams for his eczema (at least he thinks it's eczema; he's never been to a dermatologist to know for sure). He has health insurance and plenty of physician friends who would see him for free—that's not the problem.

The problem is he understands far too well how disease waits for every body, and part of him still believes that not acknowledging there's something wrong will make it go away.

My father is not unusual among his friends. They are cardiologists who smoke, psychiatrists and gynecologists who fall asleep in the middle of a mahjong and drinking binge. One colleague, a radiologist with two children under the age of six, was covered in bruises and so fatigued that she was crawling up the stairs. By the time she allowed doctors to confirm what she already knew, leukemia, she had three months to live.

Five months have passed since the question began to form in my father's mind. The tumors have grown quickly, and in that time Joli's eye has become blind. There's no guarantee doctors could have saved that eye even if they had found the cancer early, before it had detached the retina. Nor is there a guarantee that removing the eye will save Joli. What if we've waited too long and the cancer cells have burst out seeds that have crawled along her optic nerve and metastasized to her brain? Her prognosis would be poor, a survival rate of less than 10 percent.

Moments before the surgery, Liza and Jorge took a family photo, the last one of Joli with her right eye. Joli wore a yellow gown, open in the back, and thick hospital socks with rough treads. Her dense curls were unbrushed. She was looking at a balloon and crying. When her parents left her on the operating table, they asked, still unable to accept the truth, "You're sure it's my kid that has cancer?"

In the days after the surgery, the doctors will perform scans and biopsies and spinal taps. They will mine bone marrow. Soon, we'll learn they've found no sign of cancer in the other eye, and no obvious signs of spreading. Despite this good news, Joli will need chemotherapy. For easy access to her vascular system, they will embed a plastic port, like a piece of uncooked ziti, next to her left nipple. For the next six months, Joli's baby-smooth skin will be bruised from needles and raw from bandage adhesive that stays stuck for days. Within a week of her first chemotherapy treatment, her Afro will fall onto her pillow as she sleeps. She will hold her curls against her chin, and say, "I'm Daddy." All this joy and suffering will happen later.

For now, we wait in Joli's hospital room and watch the light change. When the doctor returns her to us, Joli does not speak or cry. Liza lies in the hospital bed, and Joli settles underneath her mother's breasts like an enraged squatter trying to move back inside the only home where she ever felt safe. If anyone tries to kiss or touch her, or if Liza moves, Joli shrieks like a wild animal. White bandages over her right eye protrude like a fist. We are afraid of what is and isn't underneath.

As we wait for the anesthesia to wear off, we sit in this room. We look out the window or at our books or laptop screens so we don't have to look at each other. We eat soup and drink coffee. We make excuses about why my father, the ophthalmologist, isn't here for his granddaughter's eye surgery. We understand that like all of us, he is doing the best he can.

The Art of Medicine Caregiving: The Odyssey of Becoming More Human

Arthur Kleinman

From the *Lancet*

"Let the more loving one be me."

W H Auden, The More Loving One

I LEAD HER across the living room, holding her hand behind my back, so that I can navigate the two of us between chairs, sofas, end tables, over Persian rugs, through the passageway and into the kitchen. I help her find and carefully place herself in a chair, one of four at the oval-shaped oak table. She turns the wrong way, forcing the chair outward; I push her legs around and in, under the table's edge. The sun streams through the bank of windows. The brightness of the light and its warmth, on a freezing winter's day, make her smile. She turns toward me. The uneven pupils in Joan Kleinman's green-brown eyes look above and beyond my head, searching for me face. Gently I turn her head towards me. I grin as she raises her eyebrows in recognition, shakes her long brown hair and the soft warmth of her sudden happiness lights up her still strikingly beautiful face. "Wonderful!" she whispers. "I'm a Palo Alto, a California girl. I like it warm."

I place a fork in her right hand and guide it to the poached egg in the deep bowl. I have already cut up the toast, so that I can help her spear pieces of bread and soak up the yolk. She can't find the tea cup in front of her, so I move her hand next to its handle .The Darjeeling tea glows hot and golden red in the Chinese tea cup. "Wonderful!" she again whispers.

Later, while I am trying to decide what she should wear, Joan frowns, fussing with her feet. "These nails are too long. And where are my shoes? I need to find my shoes?" She stands before about 18 pairs on a rack, shoes her unseeing brain can't recognize. "Don't get agitated," I interject with foreboding. "Do you want a Zyprexa?"

"No! No pills. Why do I need pills. I'm healthy."

"Joan, you have Alzheimer's disease. You're not healthy. You have a brain disease. A serious problem." I can barely conceal the frustration in my voice.

"Why did God do this to me? I've always been good. I never did anything to cause this. Should I kill myself?" She says it in such a way as to signal to me, as she has before, that this is a statement of pain and a cry for help, not an earnest question to discuss or to make plans. In fact it means the opposite: because, as in the past, she quickly changes tone. "If you love then you can do it! We can live and love."

"We can do it" I repeat, each time a little bit more weakly, enduring the unendurable. And so, another morning begins, another day of caregiving and care-receiving between a 67-year-old man and a 69-year-old woman who have lived together passionately and collaboratively for 43 years, absorbed in an intense relationship—intellectual, aesthetic, sexual, emotional, moral. What has made it possible to get even this far are our two adult children, their spouses, my 95-year-old mother, my brother, and our four grandchildren who sometimes take the hand of their often uncomprehending grandmother, because she is standing alone, lost, and lead her back into the protective, enable circle of our family.

For 5 years we have lived through the progressive neuro-degenerative disorder that has unspoiled the neural networks of Joan's brain. It originated in the occipital lobes at the far back of the brain. The pathology of undoing has inexorably worked its way forward to the parietal and temporal lobes on the sides of the brain, and finally to the frontal lobes that mount up behind the forehead, through the layers of neurons and nodes of connecting neural nets that structure and retain memories, focus attention, balance emotion with common sense, under-write judgment, and make possible the ordinariness of reading, writing, telling stories, understanding jokes, recognizing people, orienting oneself in space and in time, but also within emo-tional and moral coordinates, and, of course, doing things in the world.

This trail of unraveled brain structure and mounting dys-function is, in physical terms, only one of inches; yet its silent implacable wrecking creates entirely new conditions for living a life and being with others. Joan has an atypical form of Alzheim-er's disease. She is, as I write, functionally blind. She cannot find her way in our home, where she has lived since 1982. She often misinterprets those objects she does see, treating a chair as if it were a table or the floor lamp a person. Left unaccompanied, she walks into doors and has banged her legs so hard into low tables she didn't see that she has caused deep contusions. Once at our son's house, she opened a door and fell down a flight of unseen stairs, breaking her pelvis; at the onset of the disease, she ran into the street, where a pick-up truck ran over her right foot.

Joan can't, on her own, find her way out of the bedroom .yet, once safely in my hands or those of our trusted home health aide, she can walk effectively. A China scholar who translates and interprets ancient texts, she can no longer read. A wife and mother whose fierce commitment to the family was its moral backbone, she now struggles to be part of family functions and can sometimes seem impassive and cut off from us. Formerly the primary caregiver for her husband and children, she is now the care-receiver. She may no longer be who she was even 5 years ago, but her subjectivity has not so much disappeared—there is much of her personality that is still present—as altered. And that alteration has affected what had been for four decades an all-consuming relationship—our identity and orientation. I still cannot accept to treat her as if she can no longer share the sensibility and narrative we have created over four decades, and yet, more and more frequently, she can't. She is happy much of the time. It is me, the caregiver, who, more often, is sad and despairing.

She is a source of great concern to each of us, her family members, about hwo to best manage her condition. We grieve what we have lost and fear what we know lies ahead. We have each of us gone through feelings of loss, anger, and frustration. We have been marked by a special kind of pain. But we have also experienced a deepening sense of responsibility, gratitude for all that we had lived through together, love solidarity and a shared sensibility that we have resisted what is beyond our control and are, individually and collectively, more for it. This is not meant as a self-satisfying summing up—there is no final summary yet and the proper genre is tragedy, as millions who are engaged in these everyday practices know.

I am writing principally about people like me who give care to loved ones who suffer the infirmities of advanced age, serious disabilities, terminal illnesses, and the devastating consequences of such health catastrophes as stroke or dementia. Faced with these crises, family and close friends become responsible for assistance with all the practical, mundane activities of daily living: dressing, feeding, bathing, toileting, ambulating, communicating, and interfacing with the health-care system. Caregivers protect the vulnerable and dependent. To use the experience-distorting technical language: they offer cognitive, behavioural, and emotional support. And because caregiving is so tiring, and emotional draining, effective caregiving requires that caregivers themselves receive practical and emotional support.

But, to use the close experiential language of actually doing it, caregiving is also a defining moral practice. It is a practice of empathic imagination, responsibility, witnessing, and solidarity with those in great need. It is a moral practice that makes caregivers, and at times even the care-receivers, more present and thereby fully human. If the ancient Chinese perception is right that we are not born fully human, but only become so as we cultivate ourselves and our relations with others—and that we must do so in a threatening world where things often go terribly wrong and where what we are able to control is very limited—then caregiving is one of those relationships and practices of self-cultivation that makes us, even as we experience our limits and failures, more human. It completes (not absolutely, but as a kind of burnishing of what we really are—warts and all) our humanity. And if that Chinese perspective is also right (as I believe it is), when it claims that by building our humanity, we humanize the world then our own ethical cultivation at the very least fosters that of others and holds the potential, through those relationships of deepening meaning, beauty, and goodness in our experience of the world.

I am not a naïve moralist. I've had far too much experience of the demands, tensions, and downright failures of caregiving to fall into sentimentality and utopianism. Caregiving is not easy. It consumes time, energy, and financial resources. It sucks out strength and determination. It turns simple ideas of efficacy and hope into big question marks. It can amplify anguish and desperation. It can divide the self. It can bring out family conflicts. It can separate out those who care from those who can't or won't handle it. It is very difficult. It is also far more complex, uncertain, and unbounded than professional medical and nursing models suggest. I know about the moral core of caregiving not nearly so much from my professional life as a psychiatrist and medical anthropologist, nor principally from the research literature and my own studies, but primarily because of my new life of practice as the primary caregiver for Joan Kleinman.

I learned to be a caregiver by doing it, because I had to do it; it was there to do. I think this is how most people learn to be caregivers, for people who are elderly, disabled, or chronically or terminally ill. But of course this is also how parents, especially mothers, learn to care for children. My point is not so dissimilar to what William James claimed was how we learn to feel emotions: we move, we respond, we act. Our muscles (voluntary and involuntary) move. And so out of practices comes affect. And out of practices comes caregiving. We are caregivers because we practices caregiving. It is all the little concrete things I described in caring for my wife that taken together and over time constitute my caregiving, that make me a caregiver. So much depends on those concrete things: the doing, the feeling, the shadings, the symphonic complexity, the inadequacy, the living at every moment and over what can be such a long journey of the incompleteness yet the presence of a caregiver.

Perhaps Death Is Proud; More Reason to Savor Life

Theresa Brown

From the *New York Times*

AT MY JOB, people die.

That's hardly our intention, but they die nonetheless.

Usually it's at the end of a long struggle—we have done everything modern medicine can do and then some, but we can't save them. Some part of their body, usually their lungs or their heart or their liver, has become too frail to function. These are the "good deaths," the ones where the family is present and knows what to expect. Like all deaths, these deaths are difficult, but they are controlled, unsurprising, anticipated.

And then there are the other deaths: quick and rare, where life leaves a body in minutes. In my hospital these deaths are "Condition A's." The "A" stands for arrest, as in cardiac arrest, as in this patient's heart has all of a sudden stopped beating and we need to try to restart it.

I am a new nurse, and recently I had my first Condition A. My patient, a particularly nice older woman with lung cancer, had been, as we say, "fine," with no complaints but a low-grade fever she'd had off and on for a couple of days. She had come in because she was coughing up blood, a problem we had resolved, and she was set for discharge that afternoon.

After a routine assessment in the morning, I left her in the care of a nursing student and moved on to other patients, thinking I was going to have a relatively calm day. About half an hour later an aide called me: "Theresa, they need you in 1022."

I stopped what I was doing and walked over to her room. The nurse leaving the room said, "She's spitting up blood," and went to the nurses' station to call her doctor.

Inside the room I found my patient with blood spilling uncontrollably from her mouth and nose. I remembered to put on gloves, and the aide handed me a face shield. I moved closer; I put my hand on her shoulder. "Are you in any pain?" I asked, as I recall, thinking that an intestinal bleed would be more fixable than whatever this was. She shook her head no.

I looked in her eyes and saw . . . what? Panic? Fear? The abandonment of hope? Or sheer desperation? Her own blood was gurgling in her throat and I yelled to the student for a suction tool to clear it out.

The patient tried to stand up so the blood would flow into a nearby trash can, and I told her, "No, don't stand up." She sat back down, started shaking and then collapsed backward on the bed.

"Is it condition time?" asked the other nurse.

"Call the code!" I yelled. "Call the code!"

The next few moments I can only describe as surreal. I felt for a pulse and there wasn't one. I started doing CPR. On the overhead loudspeaker, a voice called out, "Condition A."

The other nurses from my floor came in with the crash cart, and I got the board. Doing CPR on a soft surface, like a bed, doesn't accomplish much; you need a hard surface to really compress the patient's chest, so every crash cart has a two-by-three-foot slab of hard fiberboard for just this purpose. I told one of the doctors to help pick her up so I could put the board under her: she was now dead weight, and heavy.

I kept doing CPR until the condition team arrived, which seemed to happen faster than I could have imagined: the intensivists—the doctors who specialize in intensive care—the I.C.U. nurses, the respiratory therapists and I'm not sure who else, maybe a pulmonologist, maybe a doctor from anesthesia.

Respiratory took over the CPR and I stood back against the wall, bloody and disbelieving. My co-workers did all the grunt work for the condition: put extra channels on her IV pump, recorded what was happening, and every now and again called out, "Patient is in asystole again," meaning she had no heartbeat.

They worked on her for half an hour. They tried to put a tube down her throat to get her some oxygen, but there was so much blood they couldn't see. Eventually they "trached" her, put a breathing hole through her neck right into her trachea, but that filled up with blood as well.

They gave her fluids and squeezed bags of epinephrine into her veins to try to get her heart to start moving. They may even have given her adenosine, a dangerous and terrifying drug that can reverse abnormal heart rythyms after briefly stopping the patient's heart.

The sad truth about a true cardiac arrest is that drugs cannot help because there is no cardiac rhythm for them to stimulate. The doctors tried anyway. They went through so many drugs that the crash cart was emptied out and runners came and went from pharmacy bringing extras.

When George Clooney and Juliana Margulies went through these routines on "E.R.," it seemed exciting and glamorous. In real life the experience is profoundly sad. In the lay vernacular of Hollywood, asystole is known as "flatlining." But my patient never had the easy narrative of the normal heartbeat that suddenly turns straight and horizontal. Her heartbeat line was wobbly and unformed, occasionally spiked in a brief run of unsynchronized beats, and at times looked regular, because chest compressions from CPR can create what looks like a real cardiac rhythm even though the patient is dead.

And my patient was dead. She had been dead when she fell back on the bed and she stayed dead through all the effort to save her, while blood and tissue bubbled out of her and the suction clogged with particles spilling from her lungs. Everyone did what she knew how to do to save her. She could not be saved.

The reigning theory was that part of her tumor had broken off and either ruptured her pulmonary artery or created a huge blockage in her heart. Apparently this can happen without warning in lung cancer patients. Only an autopsy could tell for sure, and in terms of the role I played in all this, it doesn't matter. I did the only thing I could do—all of us did—and you can't say much more than that.

I am 43. I came to nursing circuitously, following a brief career as an English professor. Often at work in the hospital I hear John Donne in my head:

> Death be not proud, though some have called thee
> Mighty and dreadful, for thou art not so.

But after my Condition A I find his words empty. My patient died looking like one of the flesh-eating zombies from "28 Weeks Later," and indeed in real life, even in the world of the hospital, a death like this is unsettling.

What can one do? Go home, love your children, try not to bicker, eat well, walk in the rain, feel the sun on your face and laugh loud and often, as much as possible, and especially at yourself. Because the only antidote to death is not poetry, or drama, or miracle drugs, or a roomful of technical expertise and good intentions. The antidote to death is life.

Fixing Mr. Fix-It: Terrible Injury Begins Personal, Physical Journey

Diane Suchetka

From the *Cleveland Plain Dealer*

PART I

NOBODY CALLS HIM Mr. Fix-it. But they wouldn't argue with you if you did.

At least they wouldn't have back then, back before February, when the accident happened, back when Norman Martin still worked as a mechanic.

For 16 years, he put in 40 hours a week at EAB Truck Service, crawling down into the concrete pits and reaching into the underbellies of cement mixers and beer trucks, ambulances and school buses. He replaced suspensions and overhauled brakes to make sure the rigs ran smoothly and the people who drove them were safe.

Trucks weren't all he fixed.

His daughter Jessica remembers as a little girl looking out the front window of their house as a car sputtered into the driveway, smoke billowing from under its hood, a stranger jumping out, calling for her father to fix whatever had gone wrong.

It happened all the time.

If Norm wasn't tinkering, he wasn't happy. He ripped up old flooring in the kitchen and put down new. He built walls in an upstairs bedroom and tore them down when his wife, Jeanie, didn't want them anymore. He adjusted brakes on the neighbor kids' bikes, cleaned the house, did the laundry.

He didn't do it to relieve Jeanie, who has a bad back and fibromyalgia. He didn't do it because she had to be up at 4 A.M. and at work at 5:30. He did it because that's the kind of guy he is.

When his niece Destany was in high school and she'd come to visit, she'd greet Norman with a few lines of that old Salt 'n' Pepa song.

"What a man, what a man, what a man

"What a mighty good man," she'd sing.

Norm would blush and walk away and she'd keep singing.

"What a man, what a man, what a man

"What a mighty good man."

Destany's got a lot of stories about Norm, about how he rescued her when her car broke down, about how he and Jeanie took her, her husband and their 1-year-old in when they fell on hard times, how Norm moved an elderly couple—old family friends—and their house full of belongings, all by himself.

He was the big, quiet guy who loved to golf, who barely spoke in a crowd. The guy you'd see biting his nails when he was nervous. The guy everybody counted on to get things done.

Then, on Feb. 29, the strangest day of the calendar, something happened that Norm Martin couldn't fix.

He was up at 5:45 that morning, a little earlier than usual, so he could get to the bank to cash his paycheck. He slid his arms through the sleeves of his gray work shirt, the one with "Norm" stitched over the pocket. He zipped up his gray work pants, tied his boots.

He knocked on his son Jake's bedroom door to wake him for school, walked down to the kitchen, put the kettle on for tea.

On the morning that it happened, Norm Martin packed his lunch, then Jake's. He washed the dishes in the sink, poured food into the dogs' bowls, grabbed his coat and walked out to the driveway to brush the half-inch of snow off his truck and his daughter's car—he always did that for Jessica.

He shoveled the driveway that morning and hopped in his green pickup, the one he'd saved for years to buy, the one he washed every week—sometimes twice—the one he refused to let anybody eat in, let alone drive. He stopped at the bank, then dropped Jake off at school and headed to the shop.

At 8, Norm Martin said good morning to the other mechanics as he walked to his pit, the one with the huge red firetruck parked over it.

A visitor might've been annoyed by the smells—engine oil and diesel exhaust. But Norm barely noticed them as he slipped off his wedding ring and tucked it away on the top shelf of his locker. He never wore it at work. If it caught on a piece of equipment, it could rip a guy's finger off.

Easy day, he thought, as he hit the green button on the two hydraulic jacks in the middle of the pit and watched them hoist the 70,000-pound firetruck up off the floor.

The truck was huge—46½ feet long, 12 feet tall, the kind you see on the news with its ladder towering over a burning building, a fireman in the bucket, hose in his hand, dousing the flames below.

Norm grabbed his tools—a wrench in his left hand, a ratchet in his right. He was better with his right, always had been. He walked down five steel steps, ducked his head under the truck's chassis and, standing in the 4-foot-deep pit, reached up with both arms to screw the dust cover back onto the brakes.

He was just about done, 19 hours into a 20-hour job. All that was left to do was to paint everything red so it looked like new.

His pit was quiet.

Over the years, Norm had trained himself to listen for warnings. Guys in his business know how metal creaks and hydraulics groan the instant before they give way. Those sounds are a mechanic's canaries, telling him to run—to get out of the hole—before something goes wrong.

They weren't there that day.

It just happened.

Pow. That's the noise the truck made when one side of it fell off its jack. The guys on the other side of the shop didn't just hear it. They felt the floor shake under their feet.

Pow.

That was it.

Norm Martin took a step back, pulled his arms toward him, looked down.

They're gone. That was his first thought. *I know they're gone.*

Blood was everywhere. Norm fell to his knees.

You've got to get out of here, the voice in his head said, *or you're going to die down here. You don't want to die.*

"Are you all right?" somebody yelled down from the shop floor.

"No," Norm yelled back. "I'm not all right."

Out of nowhere, like a giant's arms, a force pulled him to his feet again.

Mom and Dad, he thought. *They're reaching down to save me. Who else could it be?*

He made his way to the stairs and, in a daze, walked up out of the pit, blood shooting out of the two stumps where his arms had been.

At the top of the stairs, he fell again, onto one knee, then the other. Slowly, he lowered his body to the floor and rolled himself onto his back.

He could hear the guys screaming.

"Get the paramedics here. Let's go."

Then two mechanics—both Army vets, one a combat life-saver, the other trained in battlefield first aid—took over. One of them ripped off his shirt and wrapped it around one stump. The other called 9-1-1, somebody else grabbed bundles of clean shop towels and helped stop the bleeding. One guy folded a jacket into a pillow and tucked it under Norm's head. One of the vets grabbed his feet, raised them up and held them there to try to keep the blood flowing to his organs, keep him from going into shock.

Norm lay on the concrete, still and pale and calm.

Jeanie, Jessica, Jacob, he said to himself.

Jeanie, Jessica, Jacob.

Jeanie, Jessica, Jacob.

If he could just keep thinking of his family, he could hold on, he was sure. He closed his eyes so he could picture their faces.

That seemed to scare his co-workers even more.

"Hang in there, Norm," one of them pleaded. "Hang in there, buddy. Help's on the way. Open your eyes. You gotta open your eyes."

Norm followed their orders. He stared at the ceiling, tried to imagine his family's faces there. But as the sound of the sirens grew closer, he shut his eyes again.

Jeanie, Jessica, Jacob.

Jeanie, Jessica, Jacob.

Jeanie, Jessica, Jacob.

Who's going to take care of them now?

Cleveland woke to a bleak day on Feb. 29. Newscasters were reporting 20 degrees, but the low ceiling of thick, gray clouds, the snow and the wind whipping at 25 miles an hour made it feel colder.

Tiffany Contipelli barely noticed. She sat inside the dispatch room of the Cuyahoga Heights Police Department, her eyes flitting between the four computer screens on her desk and three security-camera monitors over her head.

She'd been doing this for 11 years. So she didn't flinch when the phone on her desk rang at 10:20 that morning, three hours into her shift.

"Emergency 9-1-1. Where's your emergency?" she said, her voice official but warm.

"Uh, I think he lost his arm," a man's voice on the other end answered slowly. "Something dropped down on him."

The man gave her an address and Contipelli repeated it in her this-means-business voice, the cue to her co-worker to radio for an ambulance. Now.

"And how old is this male?" Contipelli continued.

"Uh, 44, 45."

She could tell the caller was in shock, but she also knew she needed information—fast—if she was going to help the guy who'd been hurt.

"Is he conscious?"

"Uh. I'm afraid to look ma'am."

"OK listen, I need to know exactly what's going on."

"Part of a truck fell off on him."

"All right—and I need to know—is the arm severed?"

"Yes, I think so."

"And how is he doing? Is he conscious?"

Before she could get the question out, the man began to answer, talking over her.

"He's what?" she asked.

The voice slowed even more.

"Flopping around."

"All right. Try to keep him as still as possible. What are you doing to try to stop the bleeding."

"I don't remember," he said quietly. "I don't know what we're doing."

Similar calls were coming into the Independence Police Department, and a dispatcher there had sent out an ambulance, too. Within minutes, the first one was at the shop.

Two paramedics hopped out with a jump kit, the bag filled with IV equipment, bandages, airway tubes—all the basics—and rushed toward the building. One of them slipped on the ice, picked himself up and hurried in behind the other.

The dispatcher had radioed details, but they'd been doing this long enough to know you don't really know what you've got till you get there.

What they had that morning was a guy lying on the floor, bloody stumps of his arms wrapped in shirts and towels, men in work uniforms circled around him, some standing, some down on their knees.

"You guys take care of this guy," one of them told the paramedics. It was an order, not a request. "He's a good man."

Just then a second ambulance pulled up and two more paramedics rushed in, wheeling a cot. The patches on their uniforms made it clear they were from another city, but instantly they clicked with the first two guys, each taking on a job that needed to be done.

"His name is Norm," one of the workers said, as paramedics made sure the bleeding was controlled, slid a backboard underneath Norm and helped him as he scooted himself onto it.

"Bear with us," one of the paramedics told him as they wheeled him out. "This is going to be a little scary, but we're going to do the best we can."

"Are you hanging in there Norm?" another asked as three of them settled him into the back of the ambulance, checked his blood pressure, pulse and respiration and jabbed needles into his legs—they couldn't use his arms—so they could get fluid and blood into him.

"I'm still here," Norm said, soft-spoken as always, but sounding a little irritated now. "Let's go. What are we waiting for?"

Nobody answered.

They were waiting for the fourth paramedic who was still in the shop. He'd run down into the pit to look for Norm's arms.

"They're here. They're here," one of Norm's co-workers
yelled from above, when he spotted them pinned between the
truck and the concrete floor. When the paramedic came up out
of the pit, he saw guys scrambling with floor jacks and a lift truck,
trying, as fast as they could, anything to raise the firetruck.

"Let's try the outriggers," the paramedic yelled. He'd trained
as a firefighter, too, so he knew how the truck worked, knew how
they might be able to raise it up.

He ran to the front of the truck, jumped in, flipped a switch.
Then he and one of Norm's co-workers ran to the back and
began pulling levers.

Metal tubes—there are two on each side of the truck—slid
out slowly like silver legs on a fat red spider. They planted themselves on the floor and raised the truck up until it was about nine
inches off the ground.

Norm's co-worker dropped to his hands and knees, pulled
the arms—dirty and still in the sleeves of Norm's gray work
shirt—out from under the truck and handed them to the paramedic, who ran back to the ambulance cradling Norm's arms
in his. He laid the heavy limbs at Norm's feet, jumped into the
driver's seat and headed for the hospital.

In the back, the other three paramedics focused on Norm.

"You're going to be OK," one of them kept saying. "You're
going to be OK. Dude, we're taking you to the best place
around."

Jeanie, Jessica, Jacob, Norm said over and over on the slippery,
nine-mile ride. If he could just keep thinking of his family, he
could hold on, he was sure.

The ambulance pulled up to the ER at MetroHealth Medical
Center, Cleveland's only Level One Trauma Center, and all four
paramedics rushed alongside the cot as they wheeled Norm into
Trauma Bay 14.

When the guys looked up, they saw 20 doctors and nurses in
surgical masks and gowns surrounding the bed, ready to go.

Norm saw them, too. He could feel them rushing around him, hear them yelling medical terms he didn't understand, see the grave looks on their faces.

He was going to die.

He knew that for sure.

What he didn't know was that in the thousands of runs these four paramedics had made in their 76 years in the business, none of them had ever been met in an emergency room by so many people waiting to save a guy's life.

Surgical team quickly gets to work reattaching Norman Martin's arms
PART II

EVEN BEFORE NORMAN Martin arrived at MetroHealth Medical Center's Emergency Room on Feb. 29, the trauma team was getting ready to save him.

Dispatchers had radioed that he was on his way. Pagers went off and the call went out: Category 1 trauma, the worst possible kind.

As soon as he arrived, they hooked him up to monitors and IVs, unwrapped the bloody shirts from his stumps, did everything they could to stop his arms from hemorrhaging, surprised not so much by his condition but the way he said "please" and "thank you" the entire time.

In the middle of the craziness, a tiny blond woman in a surgical mask and gown stopped to talk to Norm.

"Can you tell us your wife's phone number?" Patty Wilcze-wski asked.

Matter-of-factly, Norm rattled off his home number.

A few minutes later, she was back.

"We can't get an answer."

Norm remembered that Jeanie was at work.

"Here's my phone," he said, trying to reach the one he kept clipped to his belt.

Then he remembered he had no way to reach it.

"Look at my cell," he told the woman. "I should still have it on me. It should have her work number in it."

He raised his head up off the hospital bed to see what was going on. Another woman, standing at his feet with scissors, was cutting off his clothes.

Then everything went black.

Kevin Malone wasn't supposed to be at MetroHealth that morning.

The hand surgeon had stopped at his office to grab business cards for a meeting of orthopedic surgeons a few days later in California. While he was at the hospital, he decided to slip into the operating room. Harry Hoyen, one of his colleagues, was perform a surgery Malone had never seen before.

Malone was looking over Hoyen's shoulder when his pager went off. It was one of his residents.

"I know you're not on call," the resident told him. "But I have a feeling you're going to be needed to help out with this."

About the same time, plastic surgeon Bram Kaufman, who had finished his first hand surgery of the day, walked out to the OR's front desk.

"Did you hear?" somebody asked. "There's a guy coming in with both arms cut off?"

"Interesting," Kaufman said. "I'm on call."

Together, he and Malone rode the elevator down to the ER.

They could see the patient was in good hands, so they headed to the adjoining trauma bay, where two black plastic garbage bags lay on the bed.

Inside each bag, a bloody arm rested on a layer of ice cubes.

Somebody knew to get them on ice.

Good.

And the cuts were pretty clean.

Good again.

Even though the bones had splintered and those splinters had splayed out like limbs on a tree, they hadn't been pulverized like they are in so many accidents.

Kaufman and Malone were almost certain they could save the left arm. It had been amputated about halfway between the hand and the elbow. It would take months, but if all went well, this guy would have some use of that hand. But it would never be normal again.

The right arm was more complicated. It had been severed at the shoulder. They knew they could reattach it, but the patient might never regain use of it.

In the best cases, nerves regenerate a few inches a year. That growth is critical. Without nerves, muscles won't work, and if they don't work, the limb won't work.

In this guy's case, it would take months just to get enough nerve regrowth for him to be able to bend his right elbow—if he was lucky. And chances were, he'd never be able to move the fingers on that hand.

And, if things didn't go well?

The doctors knew they could always go back into surgery, remove the arm and fit him with a prosthesis.

After a few minutes of discussion, Kaufman made the call.

"It's a go," he said. They'd try to reattach both.

He and Malone headed to the OR, as nurses gathered saws and drills and metal plates and screws and scalpels and retractors and forceps—all wrapped in sterilized cloth—and ran them into the operating room. Inside, other nurses unwrapped them and set them up within easy reach of the doctors.

Then Norm was wheeled in and nurses wiped him down with antiseptic. Anesthesiologists hooked him up to a breathing machine and started an IV so they could give him the massive amounts of blood and other fluids he'd need to stay alive.

And at 11:20 A.M., an hour after Norman Martin lost his limbs, more than 20 doctors and nurses began putting him back together again.

It was tunnel vision from then on—doctors and nurses and residents calling on years of schooling and experience, focused on nothing but getting the job done.

Malone, wearing glasses with built-in microscopes, started by cutting off damaged skin and muscle, then bone, on the stump of Norm's left arm.

On a back table, Kaufman worked on the severed end, doing the same.

As he did, Hoyen, who'd just finished surgery, walked past the OR. A physician's assistant stopped him.

"You have to come into this room," the PA told him. "They have a big emergency."

Hoyen walked in and immediately began work on the right stump, heading the team there.

On the left, Malone's team reattached the bone with metal plates and screws. Then, with sutures as fine as human hair, they stitched arteries and veins back together again.

Three hours after the surgery began, blood was flowing into the left hand.

Twenty minutes later, Hoyen's team had it flowing into the right.

There were hours of work after that—reconnecting muscle and tendons and skin.

Each doctor left, one by one, as his job was done.

At 6:30 P.M., the surgery was over.

Kaufman was elated, but running through his mind was a list of things he needed to do next. Still in scrubs, he walked into the surgical waiting room, packed with people, their cell phones ringing, empty pizza boxes on the tables beside them.

Norm's wife, Jeanie; their children, Jessica and Jake; and other family members gathered around Kaufman, with tears in their eyes.

"Things went well," he told them. "We have the arms reattached. But we have things to worry about.

"All we've really done," he said, "is get the blood flowing. That's a big step. But we're nowhere near saving his arms at this point."

Jeanie listened and nodded as tears dripped down her face.

She stayed at Norm's side for hours that night as visitors streamed in and out of his room.

They don't let all these people into intensive care, she thought. This only happens when someone's dying.

Finally, at 2 in the morning, she went home, crawled into bed and lay awake wondering how she was going to live without the only man she'd ever loved.

Wife becomes his caregiver after accident
PART III

THEY MET WHEN she was 12 and he was 16.

Four years later, Jeanie Cimbulic and Norman Martin were married, and four years after that their daughter, Jessica, was born.

Their son, Jacob, followed 4½ years after that.

Jeanie's sisters and friends were always telling her how lucky she was to have a husband who did the dishes, took the kids to doctors' appointments, roasted the turkey every Thanksgiving.

She knew they were right.

With her fibromyalgia and bad back, she never would have survived without him.

Then the accident happened.

Norm would've never made it if not for his co-workers and the paramedics, doctors and nurses. But Jeanie, she put in more hours than all of them together.

She was his aide. She gave him baths and tucked in the blankets he kicked off while he slept.

She was his cheerleader. She celebrated every surgery he made it through and pushed him to keep going after the excitement of being alive faded and depression—over how little he could do—took its place.

She was his cook. She made bacon and eggs or pancakes and sausage and delivered them to his room so he wouldn't have to eat those hospital breakfasts.

She was his security guard. She kept people away so Norm wouldn't be embarrassed by what he could no longer do.

And she was his arms. She pushed the call button when he needed more pain medication or a nurse, changed the TV channels, helped him use the bathroom.

And she made it all look easy, even in the beginning, when just looking at Norm's arms was work.

The half-beast, half-superhero limbs were so swollen they reminded you of the Incredible Hulk, so covered in stitches they reminded you of Frankenstein's monster.

And the right one, the one he'd lost at the shoulder, caused him so much pain when he stood, he wasn't walking nearly as often as he should've been.

So Jeanie became his drill sergeant, too.

"You're going to start getting up and walking whether you like it or not," she told him one day in March.

"Why are you being so mean to me?" he asked.

"So you can come home."

Those were the magic words.

After that, Norm walked even though it took Jeanie and two other people to help him down the hospital hall. One stood behind him, in case he fell. One stood on his left to hold the pump that drew fluid off his arm. And Jeanie stood on his right, held that arm so the weight of it wouldn't pull on his shoulder, so he could avoid the worst pain of the whole ordeal, the feeling that someone was trying to pull off his arm.

He came out of his funk a bit after that, started using one of his favorite lines.

"All I want to do," he'd say with a shrug and a smile, "is be able to drive my truck and zip up my pants."

But he also started asking himself why.

Why me? Why did this happen to me?

It was a question nobody could answer.

On April 8, Dr. Bram Kaufman stopped by his hospital room and told him he'd made enough progress. The next day—40 days after the accident—Norm went home.

That made life harder for Jeanie.

Norm was still attached to a pump that drained fluid off his left arm, was still hooked up to IV antibiotics. He could barely move the fingers on his left hand, couldn't move them at all on his right. Both arms were wrapped in gauze and covered with elastic bandages to keep the swelling down, then strapped into braces to stop his fingers from curling in like claws.

Jeanie had to do everything for him.

She was up every night, once to replace the IV bag of antibiotics that dripped into his body 24 hours a day, twice more to drop pain pills into his mouth, feeding him crackers first so he wouldn't get sick.

No matter how little sleep she got, she had to be out of bed for good at 6, to get Jake up for school and Norm ready for the day.

She got him dressed, made his breakfast, fed it to him bite by bite, wiped his chin when he was done.

Then—on the five days a week the home health nurse didn't come—she re-dressed Norm's wounds, unhooking the braces, unwinding the elastic bandages, unwrapping the layers of gauze. Then wrapping his arms back up with clean bandages.

On a good day, it took 30 minutes.

And she still had to massage his fingers, one knuckle at a time, to keep them from clawing.

That took another two hours.

If she was lucky, she'd get herself a shower. Then she'd throw on her clothes and get them both out the door by 9:30 A.M., to make it to MetroHealth Medical Center by 10, for the first of Norm's string of appointments.

There were sessions with occupational therapists, physical therapists, orthopedic and plastic surgeons, an infectious disease specialist. Some days there were tests, too, and stops at the drugstore to refill prescriptions.

They'd pull back into their driveway at 1:30 or 2, when Jeanie would make lunch and feed Norm in between grabbing a few bites herself, doing the dishes and laundry and starting dinner.

She had to get that on the table for the kids and get Norm fed by 6:30. That's when she headed out to her part-time job— taking care of an elderly woman with multiple sclerosis—to help pay the bills.

Before she left, she made sure one of the kids or one of her sisters could stay with Norm, in case something went wrong and he needed help.

She was back at 9:30 to start her evening routine.

She'd re-dress Norm's wounds, go through his stretching exercises if she hadn't done them earlier, do the dishes, throw in another load of laundry, tidy the house, feed the dogs and let them out, and get Norm upstairs and into bed, dropping his evening pills into his mouth, propping pillows under his arms.

On the days she couldn't handle any more, she'd tell the kids to keep an eye on their father and she'd drive 20 minutes to her sister Kim's house, sit at the kitchen table with a cup of coffee and—she'd never tell Norm this—cry.

Then she'd drive back home to put herself to bed.

Sometimes it was 11 at night when she got home. But Norm was always up.

With her lying next to him, he'd tell her the story of the accident again, beginning to end. He needed to get it out. It was the same story every night, but as each day passed, Norm was able to let out a few more details he'd kept to himself.

"It could've been worse," he said one night as summer was coming to an end.

He repeated it a few nights later, then again a few nights after that.

"What do you keep saying that for?" Jeanie finally asked.

Norm looked up at the ceiling, took a deep breath, heard his voice crack as he answered.

Seconds before the truck fell, Norm told her, his head had been exactly where his hands were.

Jeanie swallowed hard, fought back tears.

And, like she did every night, she fluffed Norm's pillows, tucked in his blanket, snuggled as close to him as she could without hurting him, kissed him all over his face, just to aggravate him and get him to laugh.

That helped her, too. It got her mind off the bills that were piling up on the dining room table—the ones she knew were about to shake up their lives even more.

Mounting bills take a toll on the family's finances PART IV

THE MONEY PROBLEMS started the minute the accident happened.

"Just take me off the schedule," Jeanie Martin told her boss when she called from the hospital waiting room, where she sat in a daze, not knowing if doctors could reattach her husband's arms or even if they could save his life.

"Don't put me back on. I don't know what's going to happen."

If Norman Martin pulled through this, there was no way his wife was leaving his side. There wasn't anything she wouldn't do—money or no money—to get him back on his feet.

She and Norm had unused vacation time, so paychecks kept coming for a few weeks.

After that, Jeanie's income dropped to zero. She lost her health insurance, too. Workers' compensation covered Norm's medical expenses, but it only paid two-thirds of his salary.

Their income was a third of what it had been before.

So on the advice of family, Jeanie called a lawyer. If they sued and won, they might have enough money to dig themselves out of this hole.

From the beginning, their attorney made one thing clear: The case could take years.

"There aren't any guarantees," he said.

Everyone involved would be looking to blame somebody else—including Norm—for what happened, the lawyer explained as he started work on the case. They had to brace themselves for that.

Three weeks after the accident, while Norm was still in the hospital, Jeanie picked up a part-time job, an hour and a half a night, caring for an elderly woman with multiple sclerosis. It brought in about $130 a week before taxes, enough to pay for hospital parking and gas.

She took a day off from taking care of Norm and drove to the welfare office to try to get help. The state would provide Medicaid coverage for their son Jake, because he was under 18, but not for his older sister Jessica or his mom.

That meant the three medications Jeanie took for fibromyalgia and high cholesterol weren't covered any more. So she stopped taking them.

"Are we going to be living in my truck?" Norm would ask her, feeling guilty for not being able to support his family.

"Don't be ridiculous," Jeanie would tell him with a wink and a smile. "We can't fit in your truck. We'll have to live in my car."

Their niece Destany was bugging them to let her throw a fund-raiser.

No way, Norm and Jeanie told her. We weren't raised that way. We don't take. We give.

"It's payback time," Destany said. She told Jeanie a story she'd read about a woman who had learned the gift of receiving one Christmas when presents magically appeared on her front porch.

"You need to learn the gift of receiving," she said.

Then she called family and friends and created "Team Norman."

Because Norm loved his Ford pickup so much, they borrowed the car maker's theme. They plastered "Norman Is Built Ford Tough" on buttons, banners and centerpieces all over a hall on Cleveland's West Side. Hundreds of friends and relatives packed the place on a Friday night in April, two months after the accident, 16 days after Norm left the hospital.

The room was lined with 6-foot-long folding tables—11 of them—covered with dozens of gift baskets loaded with donated items.

Golf balls and tees and free passes to a local course filled one. Another overflowed with pasta, jars of sauce and breadsticks.

Somebody had crocheted a pink and blue baby blanket. A local artist donated one of her paintings. The Browns gave a jersey. The Indians, an autographed photo of Casey Blake.

The band played for free.

The owners of the hall offered that up, too.

And then there was the food—tables covered with meat platters and cookie trays and pizza and chicken wings.

The room filled with cousins and second cousins and guys Norm had gone to elementary school with, all of them talking about his big heart, how he didn't have a mean bone in his body, how something like this should never happen to such a nice guy.

They joked and laughed. But you could see their nervousness—about seeing Norm, about what to say—underneath it all. When Norm finally showed up, his eyes searched the floor, he bit his lip and, with both arms swaddled in bandages and cradled in slings, he gingerly made his way to a table in the middle of the room.

One by one, friends stopped by to say hello, to hug his neck, tousle his hair, do their best to shake his good hand, the one he could barely use.

"How you doing?" they'd ask.

"Hanging in there," Norm would tell them with a closed-lipped smile and a nod, his right knee bouncing nonstop now that he couldn't bite his nails.

No one lingered. And at times, it seemed Norm was a stranger at his own party.

"Thank God he has his arms back," somebody said. "At least he can hug his wife and children."

The band played "Sweet Home Alabama," "Johnny B. Good" and "Blue Suede Shoes." In between songs, Destany and other members of Team Norman took to the microphone and auctioned off the baskets.

Jeanie sat at Norm's side, cut food from her plate and fed it to him while a man across the table did the exact same thing to his 15-month-old granddaughter.

As the night wore on, couples began to dance between the tables and a guy in the band moved to the microphone. "Come on everybody," he yelled, "put your hands together."

Nobody flinched. Not even Norm.

After expenses, Destany handed her aunt and uncle $9,500.

Jeanie bought Norm some new clothes. He'd lost so much weight, his old ones didn't fit. She got caught up on her car payments, the utilities, the credit cards.

She dipped into the money to put a new roof on the house. The old one was falling apart. A friend put it on for free, with Jake's help. And Norm stood back, barely able to watch, sick that he couldn't do the work himself.

As the weeks went by, Jeanie had no choice but to start using the money for groceries, too. By September, it was spent.

Collection agencies called so frequently, she swore she was going to have her phone disconnected. And with winter a few months away, she knew she finally had to make the call she'd been putting off.

On a late summer day, a real estate agent pounded a For Sale sign into their front yard.

They'd sell the house before the bank foreclosed, move into an apartment with no grass to cut and a maintenance man to fix all the things Norm could not.

They found a place right away, across the street from Jeanie's sister.

Now, if they need help, family can be there in a few minutes. Rent's not so bad. With their daughter Jessica living on her own, they only need two bedrooms.

But anything beyond the basics, they can't afford.

Jake needs a winter coat.

And, as Jeanie says, "Christmas ain't happening this year."

Something better is.

Still recovering himself, Norm turns focus to others
PART V

IT'S TAKEN A lot more than doctors and nurses and family and friends to get Norman Martin where he is today.

The list of people who've helped is long. And the name at the top is Norman Martin.

"He's as hard-working a patient as I've ever had," his physical therapist, Tim Walsh, said just before Thanksgiving, as he went over Norm's chart.

"Honestly, all the gains this guy's had are because he's a workhorse."

His doctors agree.

"There are people who smash their little finger and feel like their life is over and they can't do anything because it hurts or it doesn't bend and they just want it back the way it was," says Bram Kaufman, one of the surgeons who reattached Norm's arms. "Then, on the other end of the spectrum, there are people like Norm. He's made tremendous progress, and most—90 percent of it—is what he's done."

His right arm still hangs like a sandbag at his side, barely usable. His left is better. Both ache all the time, the kind of throbbing you feel after you've hammered your thumb.

But he's determined to regain as much use of both of them as he can.

He goes to physical and occupational therapy twice a week. He works out at home with exercise bands. He walks a mile every day that there's no snow or ice to trip him up. Even when he's sitting in his recliner, watching football or old John Wayne movies, he stretches his shoulder, flexes his biceps, grips whatever he can with his left hand to build strength in it.

Those who've worked with him in the 10 months since the accident are awed by his progress—and his luck.

"The stars were aligned," says Patty Wilczewski, the trauma coordinator who helped Norm after paramedics rushed him into the emergency room.

"If this would've happened at 9 o'clock at night," says orthopedic surgeon Harry Hoyen, "we would not have been able to mobilize enough people to save both arms. It wouldn't have happened."

It wouldn't have happened if two of Norm's co-workers hadn't been Army vets trained in first aid.

It wouldn't have happened if the paramedics hadn't been trained as firefighters, if one of them hadn't been there to raise up the firetruck.

It wouldn't have happened if Dr. Kevin Malone hadn't stopped by MetroHealth Medical Center to pick up some business cards, or Hoyen hadn't been walking by the operating room shortly after the surgery began.

And, it wouldn't have happened if Norm wasn't so intent on making it happen.

"My dad's the kind of person, he won't give up," says his son, Jake. "I'm so proud of him."

"He just makes me proud that I was able to help him," says Duane Kattler, one of the paramedics who rescued him.

"He's a master fixer-upper," says his rehabilitation psychologist, Elizabeth Dreben.

"A living miracle," says his niece Destany.

"And he's not done," says his daughter, Jessica. "There's more to come."

"I have a feeling we're all going to get surprised by it," his wife, Jeanie, says.

A month after the accident, Norm started telling people, with a laugh, that all he wanted to do was drive his truck and zip up his pants. Back then it was tough for him to imagine doing either.

No matter how hard he tried to squeeze his good hand—the left—into a fist in those days, he could never get his thumb and fingers more than three inches apart.

Then, in May, he picked up a kitchen sponge with that hand.

In June, his occupational therapist handed him a pen and asked him to try using it. He wrote his name.

A few weeks ago, Jeanie got out his golf clubs and Norm started putting balls around the house.

On Thanksgiving morning, she strapped a special brace on his hand, and he shaved himself. He's carried a few electric tools in from the garage and he's recharging them. And when his nephew and brother-in-law tried to fix his truck, Norm went outside and helped diagnose the problem.

He can throw his right arm over Jeanie's shoulder now, reach around her waist with the left, and hug her.

He's laughing more, too, poking fun at himself.

With a special pull, he may be able to zip up his pants pretty soon.

And with an occupational therapist in the passenger seat of a specially equipped van, he's been driving around town like there's nothing wrong with his arms at all.

Today, at 3:30 he'll take his driver's test in that van. If he passes, he'll have his license back. He won't have to depend on Jeanie or Jessica to drive him around.

And in January, doctors are going to take him into surgery again—for the 23rd time since the accident—to transplant a nerve from his leg into his right arm in the hopes that he'll be able to bend that wrist, maybe one day use his fingers a bit on that hand.

That's the progress his body is making.

His head has made even more.

Not long after Dreben began seeing Norm, she gave him the talk she gives most of her patients.

"You're still you," the rehabilitation psychologist told him, waving her hands with enthusiasm. "The disability isn't running the show. Your identity—who you are as a human being—doesn't reside in that paralyzed arm or that missing leg. You're not your missing arms. You're a valuable human being. You're still you in there."

Yeah, right.

That's what Norm thought in the beginning.

He knows better now.

He's not his disability.

He's still the same guy he always was, the guy who takes care of everybody else, the guy who can't help but fix what needs to be fixed.

What needs fixing now, he says, is workplace safety.

Let the lawyers fight it out over who's to blame for what happened to him.

He's staying away from that. He's looking ahead instead.

"I don't want this to happen to anybody else," he says, shaking his head back and forth, looking down at his bandaged arms. "I would never want to see anybody's family going through what mine is going through right now."

Jeanie looks up at him. Tells him he's no trouble. That he would do the same for any of them. But Norm doesn't seem to hear her.

"Maybe I could go out to companies, talk about safety," he says. "That would make me feel a lot better, knowing that I'm keeping other people from getting hurt."

He's quiet for a bit after that. Then he starts again.

"If I can help one person," he says. "If I can just help one person."

Nobody calls him Mr. Fix-it.

But after all this, maybe they'll start.

Norman Martin, 'Mr. Fix-it,' passes his driver's test

NORMAN MARTIN TOSSED and turned all night Wednesday.

The restlessness didn't come from the throbbing pain in his reattached arms or nightmares of the accident that severed them nearly 10 months ago.

The 46-year-old truck mechanic was worried about something he hadn't thought about in years: passing his driving test.

With his wife, Jeanie, and his children, Jessica and Jacob, waiting, he passed—without any trouble—Thursday afternoon.

A little after 4 P.M., he left an Ohio Bureau of Motor Vehicles exam station with his driver's license in his wife's hand and a smile on his face.

To be licensed, he had to prove he could drive a specially equipped van safely, despite the limited use of his hands. He won't be able to drive his beloved green pickup truck again until it's outfitted with similar equipment.

That's weeks away.

But once it's done, he's hitting the road.

"I think I'm just going to drive," he said, pausing for a moment, "until the tires fall off."

The *Plain Dealer* has been telling the story of Norman Martin's accident and recovery in a series titled "Fixing Mr. Fix-It."

Since it began Sunday, more than 150 readers—from Cleveland to Chicago to North Carolina—have e-mailed and called the newspaper to ask how to help the family. They lost their home and have struggled financially since Feb. 29, the day a 70,000-pound firetruck that Norm Martin was fixing at work fell on him and cut off one arm and much of the other.

A team of more than 20 doctors and nurses reattached his arms that day. And he's been working ever since to regain the use of them.

This week, employees of several businesses called to say they were taking up collections for food, clothing and presents.

One man offered a job. Another said he could provide special golf lessons for people with disabilities. A third anonymously sent a check for $10,000.

"Oh my gosh," Jeanie Martin cried, when she heard about the generous donations. "My kids can have a Christmas."

The Martins have expressed their gratitude, over and over, to everyone who's helped them in any way.

"We feel so blessed that people we don't know are so willing to help," Jeanie Martin said Thursday. "Though it was not expected, it certainly is appreciated. Thank you and God bless."

Norm Martin said thanks, too, to the dozens of people who saved his life—from co-workers Jim Lee and Ed Taraska, who applied their Army first aid immediately after the accident, to the Valley View and Independence paramedics who rushed him to the hospital, to the doctors, nurses and therapists who cared for him during and after his 40-day stay at MetroHealth Medical Center.

"I'm just grateful to them and their hard work and dedica-
tion to help get through everything," he said Thursday night.
"The paramedics, my co-workers, they just did a great job. And
I would do the same for any one of them."

A Summer of Madness

Oliver Sacks

From the *New York Review of Books*

"ON JULY 5, 1996," Michael Greenberg starts, "my daughter was struck mad." No time is wasted on preliminaries, and *Hurry Down Sunshine* moves swiftly, almost torrentially, from this opening sentence, in tandem with the events that it tells of. The onset of mania is sudden and explosive: Sally, the fifteen-year-old daughter, has been in a heightened state for some weeks, listening to Glenn Gould's Goldberg Variations on her Walkman, poring over a volume of Shakespeare's sonnets till the early hours. Greenberg writes:

> *Flipping open the book at random I find a blinding criss-cross of arrows, definitions, circled words. Sonnet 13 looks like a page from the Talmud, the margins crowded with so much*

commentary the original text is little more than a speck at the center.

Sally has also been writing singular, Sylvia Plath–like poems. Her father surreptitiously glances at these, finds them strange, but it does not occur to him that her mood or activity is in any way pathological. She has had learning difficulties from an early age, but she is now triumphing over these, finding her intellectual powers for the first time. Such exaltation is normal in a highly gifted fifteen-year-old. Or so it seems.

But, on that hot July day, she breaks—haranguing strangers in the street, demanding their attention, shaking them, and then suddenly running full tilt into a stream of traffic, convinced she can bring it to a halt by sheer willpower (with quick reflexes, a friend yanks her out of the way just in time).

Robert Lowell described something very similar in an attack of "pathological enthusiasm":

> *The night before I was locked up I ran about the streets of Bloomington Indiana.... I believed I could stop cars and paralyze their forces by merely standing in the middle of the highway with my arms outspread.*

Such sudden, dangerous exaltations and actions are not uncommon at the start of a manic attack.

Lowell had a vision of Evil in the world, and of himself, in his "enthusiasm," as the Holy Ghost. Sally had, in some ways, an analogous vision of moral collapse, seeing all around her the loss or suppression of God-given "genius," and of her own mission to help everyone reclaim that lost birthright. That it was such a vision which led to her passionate confrontation with strangers, her bizarre behavior imbued with a sense of her own special powers, her parents learn when they quiz her the next day:

She has had a vision. It came to her a few days ago, in the Bleecker Street playground, while she was watching two little girls play on the wooden footbridge near the slide. In a surge of insight she saw their genius, their limitless native little-girl genius, and simultaneously realized that we are all geniuses, that the very idea the word stands for has been distorted. Genius is not the fluke they want us to believe it is, no, it's as basic to who we are as our sense of love, of God. Genius is childhood. The Creator gives it to us with life, and society drums it out of us before we have the chance to follow the impulses of our naturally creative souls . . . .

Sally related her vision to the little girls in the playground. Apparently they understood her perfectly. Then she walked out onto Bleecker Street and discovered her life had changed. The flowers in front of the Korean deli in their green plastic vases, the magazine covers in the news shop window, the buildings, cars—all took on a sharpness beyond anything she had imagined. The sharpness, she said, "of present time." A wavelet of energy swelled through the center of her being. She could see the hidden life in things, their detailed brilliance, the funneled genius that went into making them what they are.

Sharpest of all was the misery on the faces of the people she passed. She tried to explain her vision to them but they just kept rushing by. Then it hit her: they already know about their genius, it isn't a secret, but much worse: genius has been suppressed in them, as it had been suppressed in her. And the enormous effort required to keep it from percolating to the surface and reasserting its glorious hold on our lives is the cause of all human suffering. Suffering that Sally, with this epiphany, has been chosen among all people to cure.

As startling as Sally's passionate new beliefs are, her father and stepmother are even more struck by her manner of speaking:

> Pat and I are dumbstruck, less by what she is saying than how she is saying it. No sooner does one thought come galloping out of her mouth than another overtakes it, producing a pile-up

of words without sequence, each sentence canceling out the pre-
vious one before it's had a chance to emerge. Our pulses racing,
we strain to absorb the sheer volume of energy pouring from her
tiny body. She jabs at the air, thrusts out her chin . . . her drive to
communicate is so powerful it's tormenting her. Each individual
word is like a toxin she must expel from her body.

The longer she speaks, the more incoherent she becomes,
and the more incoherent she becomes, the more urgent is her
need to make us understand her! I feel helpless watching her.
And yet I am galvanized by her sheer aliveness.

One may call it mania, madness, or psychosis—a chemical
imbalance in the brain—but it presents itself as energy of a primor-
dial sort. Greenberg likens it to "being in the presence of a rare
force of nature, such as a great blizzard or flood: destructive, but in
its way astounding too." Such unbridled energy can resemble that
of creativity or inspiration or genius—this, indeed, is what Sally
feels is rushing through her—not an illness, but the apotheosis of
health, the release of a deep, previously suppressed self.

These are the paradoxes that surround what Hughlings Jack-
son, the nineteenth-century neurologist, called "super-positive"
states: they betoken disorder, imbalance in the nervous system,
but their energy, their euphoria, makes them feel like supreme
health. Some patients may achieve a startled insight into this,
as did one patient of mine, a very old lady with neurosyphilis.
Becoming more and more vivacious in her early nineties, she
said to herself, "You're feeling too well, you must be ill." George
Eliot, similarly, spoke of herself as feeling "dangerously well"
before the onset of her migraine attacks.

Mania is a biological condition that feels like a psychological one—a state of mind. In this way it resembles the effects of
various intoxications. I saw this very dramatically with some
of my *Awakenings* patients when they began taking L-dopa, a
drug which is converted in the brain to the neuro-transmitter
dopamine. Leonard L., in particular, became quite manic on

this: "With L-dopa in my blood," he wrote at the time, "there's nothing in the world I can't do if I want." He called dopamine "resurrectamine" and started to see himself as a messiah—he felt that the world was polluted with sin and that he had been called upon to save it. And in nineteen nonstop, almost sleepless days and nights, he typed an entire autobiography of 50,000 words. "Is it the medicine I am taking," wrote another patient, "or just my new state of mind?"

If there is uncertainty in a patient's mind about what is "physical" and what is "mental," there may be a still deeper uncertainty as to what is self or not-self—as with my patient Frances D., who, as she grew more excited on L-dopa, was taken over by strange passions and images which she could not dismiss as entirely alien to her "real self." Did they, she wondered, come from very deep but previously suppressed parts of herself? But these patients, unlike Sally, knew that they were on a drug, and could see, all around them, similar effects taking hold on the others.

For Sally there was no precedent, no guide. Her parents were as bewildered as she was—more so, because they did not have her mad assurance. Was it, they wondered, something she had been taking—had she dropped acid, or something worse? And if not, was it something that they had bequeathed her in their genes, or something awful they had "done" at a critical stage in her development? Was it something she had always had in her, even though it was triggered so suddenly?

These were the questions my own parents asked themselves when, in 1943, my fifteen-year-old brother Michael became acutely psychotic. My brother saw "messages" everywhere, felt his thoughts were being read or broadcast, had explosions of strange giggling, and felt he had been translocated to another "realm." Hallucinatory drugs were rare in the 1940s, so my parents, who were both doctors, wondered whether Michael might have some psychosis-producing illness—perhaps a thyroid condition or a brain tumor. It ultimately became clear, though, that my brother suffered from a schizophrenic psychosis. In Sally's case, blood tests and physical exams ruled out any problems with thyroid levels, intoxicants, or tumors. Her psychosis, though acute and dangerous (all psychoses are potentially dangerous, at least to the patient), was "merely" manic.

One can become manic—or depressed—without becoming psychotic: having delusions or hallucinations, losing sight of reality. Sally, though, did go over the top, and on that hot July day, something happened, something snapped. All of a sudden, she was a different person—she looked different, sounded different. "Suddenly every point of connection between us had vanished," her father writes. She calls him "Father" (he was "Dad" before), and speaks in a "pressured, phony voice, as if delivering stage lines she has learned"; "her normally warm chestnut eyes are shell-like and dark, as if they've been brushed over with lacquer."

Greenberg tries to speak to her of ordinary matters, asking her if she is hungry or wants to lie down:

> Each time, however, her otherness is reaffirmed. It is as if the real Sally has been kidnapped, and here in her place is a demon, like Solomon's, who has appropriated her body. The ancient superstition of possession! How else to come to grips with this grotesque transformation?
>
> . . . In the most profound sense Sally and I are strangers: we have no common language.

The special qualities of mania have been recognized and distinguished from other forms of madness since the great physicians of antiquity wrote on the subject. Aretaeus, in the second century, gave a clear description of how excited and depressed states might alternate in an individual, but the distinction between different forms of madness was not formalized until the rise of psychiatry in nineteenth-century France. It was then that "circular insanity" (*folie circulaire or folie à double forme*)—what Emil Kraepelin later called manic-depressive insanity and what we would now call bipolar disorder—was distinguished from the much graver disorder of "dementia praecox" or schizophrenia. But medical accounts, accounts from the outside, can never do justice to what is actually experienced in the course of such psychoses; there is no substitute here for firsthand accounts.

There have been several such personal accounts over the years, and one of the best, to my mind, is *Wisdom, Madness and Folly: The Philosophy of a Lunatic* by John Custance, published in 1952. He writes:

The mental disease to which I am subject is . . . known as manic depression, or, more accurately, as Manic depressive Psychosis . . . The manic state is one of elation, of pleasurable excitement sometimes attaining to an extreme pitch of ecstasy; the depressive state is its precise opposite, one of misery, dejection, and at times of appalling horror.

Custance had his first manic attack at the age of thirty-five, and would continue to have periodic episodes of mania or depression for the next twenty years:

> *When the nervous system is thoroughly deranged, the two contrasting states of mind can be almost infinitely intensified. It sometimes seems to me as though my condition had been specially devised by Providence to illustrate the Christian concepts of Heaven and Hell. Certainly it has shown me that within my own soul there are possibilities of an inner peace and happiness beyond description, as well as of inconceivable depths of terror and despair.*
>
> *Normal life and consciousness of "reality" appear to me rather like motion along a narrow strip of table-land at the top of a Great Divide separating two distinct universes from each other. On the one hand the slope is green and fertile, leading to a lovely landscape where love, joy and the infinite beauties of nature and of dreams await the traveller; on the other a barren, rocky declivity, where lurk endless horrors of distorted imagination, descends to the bottomless pit.*

In the condition of manic- depression, this table-land is so narrow that it is exceedingly difficult to keep on it. One begins to slip; the world about one changes imperceptibly. For a time it is possible to keep some sort of grip on reality. But once one is really over the edge, once the grip of reality is lost, the forces of the Unconscious take charge, and then begins what appears to be an unending voyage into the universe of bliss or the universe of horror as the case may be, a voyage over which one has oneself no control whatever.

In our own time, Kay Redfield Jamison, a brilliant and courageous psychiatrist who has manic-depressive illness herself, has written both the definitive medical monograph on this subject (*Manic-Depressive Illness, with Frederick K. Goodwin, 1990; second edition, 2007*) and a personal memoir (*An Unquiet Mind, 1995*). In the latter, she writes:

> I was a senior in high school when I had my first attack of manic-depressive illness; once the siege began, I lost my mind rather rapidly. At first, everything seemed so easy. I raced about like a crazed weasel, bubbling with plans and enthusiasms, immersed in sports, and staying up all night, night after night, out with friends, reading everything that wasn't nailed down, filling manuscript books with poems and fragments of plays, and making expansive, completely unrealistic, plans for my future. The world was filled with pleasure and promise; I felt great. Not just great, I felt really great. I felt I could do anything, that no task was too difficult. My mind seemed clear, fabulously focused, and able to make intuitive mathematical leaps that had up to that point entirely eluded me. Indeed, they elude me still.
>
> At that time, however, not only did everything make perfect sense, but it all began to fit into a marvelous kind of cosmic relatedness. My sense of enchantment with the laws of the natural world caused me to fizz over, and I found myself buttonholing my friends to tell them how beautiful it all was. They were less

*than transfixed by my insights into the webbings and beauties of
the universe, although considerably impressed by how exhausting it was to be around my enthusiastic ramblings . . . . Slow
down, Kay . . . . For God's sake, Kay, slow down.*

I did, finally, slow down. In fact, I came to a grinding halt.

Jamison contrasts this experience with the episodes that
came later:

*Unlike the very severe manic episodes that came a few years
later and escalated wildly and psychotically out of control, this
first sustained wave of mild mania was a light, lovely tincture
of true mania . . . . It was short-lived and quickly burned itself
out: tiresome to my friends, perhaps; exhausting and exhilarat-
ing to me, definitely; but not disturbingly over the top.*

Both Jamison and Custance describe how mania alters
not just thought and feeling, but even their sensory perceptions. Custance carefully itemizes these changes in his memoir.
Sometimes the electric lights in the ward have "a bright starlike
phenomenon emanat[ing] . . . ultimately forming a maze of
iridescent patterns." Faces seem to "glow with a sort of inner
light which shows up the characteristic lines extremely vividly."
Though normally "a hopeless draughtsman," Custance is able
to draw quite well while manic (I was reminded here of my own
ability to do this, many years ago, during a period of amphet-
amine-induced hypomania); all of his senses seem intensified:

*My fingers are much more sensitive and neat. Although
generally a clumsy person with an execrable handwriting I can
write much more neatly than usual; I can print, draw, embel-
lish and carry out all sorts of little manual operations, such
as pasting up scrapbooks and the like, which would normally
drive me to distraction. I also note a particular tingling in my
fingertips.*

> *My hearing appears to be more sensitive, and I am able to take in . . . many different sound-impressions at the same time . . . From the cries of gulls outside to the laughter and chatter of my fellow-patients, I am fully alive to what is going on and yet find no difficulty in concentrating on my work.*
>
> *. . . If I were to be allowed to walk about freely in a flower garden I should appreciate the scents far more than usual . . . . Even common grass tastes excellent, while real delicacies like strawberries or raspberries give ecstatic sensations appropriate to a veritable food of the gods.*

At first, Sally's parents struggle to believe (as Sally herself believes) that her excited state is something positive, something other than illness. Her mother puts a somewhat New Agey spin on it:

> *Sally is having an experience, Michael, I'm sure of it, this isn't a sickness. She's a highly spiritual girl.... What's happening right now is a necessary phase in Sally's evolution, her journey toward a higher realm.*

And this interpretation finds echoes of a more classical kind in Greenberg himself:

> *I wanted to believe this too . . . . to believe in her break-through, her victory, the delayed efflorescence of her mind. But how does one tell the difference between Plato's "divine madness" and gibberish? between [enthusiasm] and lunacy? between the prophet and the "medically mad"?*

(It was similar, Greenberg points out, with James Joyce and his schizophrenic daughter, Lucia. "Her intuitions are amazing," Joyce remarked. "Whatever spark of gift I possess has been trans-mitted to her and has kindled a fire in her brain." Later, he told

Beckett, "She's not a raving lunatic, just a poor child who tried to do too much, to understand too much.")

But it becomes clear within hours that Sally is indeed psychotic and out of control, and her parents take her to a psychiatric hospital. At first, she welcomes this, seeing the nurses, the attendants, and the psychiatrists as specially tuned to understand her insight, her message. The reality is brutally different: she is stupefied with tranquilizers and put in a locked ward.

Greenberg's description of the ward takes on the richness and density of a novel, embracing a Chekhovian cast of characters—the staff, the other patients on the ward. He sees a highly disturbed, obviously psychotic young Hasidic man, whose family will not accept that he is ill: "He has achieved *devaykah*," says his brother, "the state of constant communion with God."

There is relatively little attempt to *understand* Sally in the hospital—her mania is treated first of all as a medical condition, a disturbance of brain chemistry, to be dealt with on a neurochemical basis. Medication is crucial, even life-saving, in acute mania, which untreated can lead to exhaustion and death. Unfortunately, though, Sally does not respond to lithium, which has been invaluable for many patients with manic-depressive illness, and so her physicians have to resort to heavy tranquilizers—which damp down her exuberance and wildness but leave her stupefied and apathetic and parkinsonian for a time. Seeing his teenage daughter in this zombie-like state is almost as shocking for her father as her mania has been.

After twenty-four days of this, Sally is released—still somewhat delusional and still on strong tranquilizers—to go home, under careful and at first continuous surveillance. Outside the hospital, she establishes a crucial relationship with an exceptional therapist, who is able to approach Sally as a human being, trying to understand her thoughts and feelings. Dr. Lensing shows a disarming directness: "I bet you feel as if there's a lion inside you" are her first words to Sally.

"How did you know?" Sally is amazed, her suspicion instantly melting away. Lensing goes on to talk of mania, Sally's mania, as if it were a sort of creature, another being, inside her:

> *Lensing nimbly lowers herself into the waiting area chair next to Sally's and tells her in a tone of woman-to-woman straight talk that mania—and she refers to it as if it is a separate entity, a mutual acquaintance of theirs—mania is a glutton for attention. It craves thrills, action, it wants to keep thriving, it will do anything to live on. "Did you ever have a friend who's so exciting you want to be around her, but she leads you into disaster and in the end you wish you never met? You know the sort of person I mean: the girl who wants to go faster, who always wants more. The girl who serves herself first and screw the rest . . . . I'm just giving an example of what mania is: a greedy, charismatic person who pretends to be your friend."*

Lensing tries to get Sally to distinguish her psychosis from her true identity, to stand outside the psychosis and to see the complex, ambiguous relationship between it and her. (Psychosis is "not an identity," she says sharply.) She speaks of this to Sally's father, too—for his understanding is also necessary if Sally is to get better. She emphasizes the seductive power of psychosis:

> *Sally . . . doesn't want to be isolated, her impulse is outward, which I can tell you is extremely good news. Her desire is to be understood, and not only by us, she wants to understand herself as well. She's still attached to her mania, of course. She's remembering the intensity of her experience, and she's doing her damnedest to keep that intensity alive. She thinks that if she gives it up, she'll lose the great abilities she believes she's acquired. It's a terrible paradox really: the mind falls in love with psychosis. The evil seduction, I call it.*

"Seduction" is the crucial word here (it is also the key word in the title of Edward Podvoll's marvelous book *The Seduction of Madness*, on the nature and treatment of mental illness). Why should psychosis, and mania in particular, be seductive? Freud spoke of all psychoses as narcissistic disorders: one becomes the most important person in the world, chosen for a unique role, whether it is to be a messiah, a redeemer of souls, or (as happens in depressive or paranoid psychoses) to be the focus of universal persecution and accusation, or derision and degradation.

But even short of such messianic feelings, mania can fill one with a sense of enormous pleasure, even ecstasy—and the sheer intensity of this may make it difficult to "give up." It is what prompts Custance, despite his knowledge of how danger-ous such a course is, to avoid medication and hospitalization in one attack of mania, and instead embrace it, undertaking a risky and rather James Bond–like adventure in East Berlin. Perhaps a similar intensity of feeling is sought by drug addicts, especially those addicted to stimulants like cocaine or amphetamines; and here, too, a high is likely to be followed by a crash, just as a mania is usually followed by a depression—both, perhaps, due to the exhaustion caused by neurotransmitters like dopamine in the overstimulated reward systems in the brain.

Mania, though, is by no means all pleasure, as Greenberg continually observes. He speaks of Sally's "pitiless ball of fire," her "terrified grandiosity," of how anxious and fragile she is inside the "hollow exuberance" of her mania. When one ascends to the exorbitant heights of mania, one becomes very isolated from ordinary human relationships, human scale—even though this isolation may be covered over by a defensive imperiousness or grandiosity. This is why Lensing sees Sally's returning desire to make genuine contact with others, to understand and be understood, as a propitious sign of her returning to health, her coming back to earth.

Psychosis, as Lensing says, is not an identity, but a temporary aberration or departure from identity. And yet having a chronic or recurring mind-altering condition like manic-depressive illness is bound to influence one's identity, to become part of one's attitudes and ways of thinking. As Jamison writes,

It is, after all, not just an illness, but something that affects every aspect of my life: my moods, my temperament, my work, and my reactions to almost everything that comes my way.

Nor is it just a piece of biological bad luck for which there is nothing to be said. Although Jamison says there is nothing good to be said for depression, she does feel that her manias and hypomanias, when not too out of control, have played a crucial and sometimes positive part in her life. Indeed, in her book *Touched with Fire: Manic-Depressive Illness and the Artistic Temperament* (1993), she has provided much evidence to suggest a possible relationship between mania and creativity, citing the many great artists—Schumann, Coleridge, Byron, and Van Gogh among them—who seem to have lived with manic-depressive illness.

When Sally is hospitalized, her father asks the psychiatric resident about her diagnosis. "Sally's condition," the resident says, "has probably been building for a while, gathering strength until it just overwhelmed her." Greenberg asks what her "condition" is:

What we call [it] is not what's important right now. Certainly many of the criteria for bipolar I are here. But fifteen is relatively early for fulminating mania to present itself.

In the last couple of decades, the term "bipolar disorder" has come into use, in part, Jamison suggests, because it is felt to be less stigmatizing than "manic-depressive illness." But, she cautions,

Splitting mood disorders into bipolar and unipolar categories presupposes a distinction between depression and manic-depressive illness . . . that is not always clear, nor supported *by science. Likewise, it perpetuates the notion that depression exists rather tidily segregated on its own pole, while mania clusters off neatly and discreetly on another. This polarization...flies in the face of everything that we know about the cauldronous, fluctuating nature of manic-depressive illness.*

Moreover, "bipolarity" is characteristic of many disorders of control—like catatonia or parkinsonism—where patients lose the middle ground of normality and alternate between hyperkinetic and akinetic states. Even in a metabolic disease such as diabetes, there may be dramatic alternations between (for instance) very high blood sugar and very low blood sugar, as the complex homeostatic mechanisms are compromised.

There is another reason why the notion of manic-depressive illness as a bipolar illness, swinging from one pole to the other, can be misleading. This was brought out by Kraepelin more than a century ago, when he wrote of "mixed states," states in which there are elements of both mania and depression, inseparably intertwined. He wrote of "the deep inward relationship of such apparently contradictory states."

We speak of "poles apart," but the poles of mania and depression are so close to each other that one wonders if depression may be a form of mania, or vice versa. (Such a dynamic notion of mania and depression—their "clinical unity," as Kraepelin put it—is underlined by the fact that lithium, for those patients in whom it works, works equally well on *both* states.) This paradoxical situation is described by Greenberg with often astonishing oxymorons, as when he speaks of the "abysmal elation" Sally sometimes feels "in the throes of [her] dystopic mania."

Sally's final return from the mad heights of her mania is almost as sudden as her taking off into it seven weeks earlier, as Greenberg recounts:

Sally and I are standing in the kitchen. I have spent the day at home with her, working on my script for Jean-Paul.

"Would you like a cup of tea?" I ask.

"That would be nice. Yes. Thank you."

"With milk?"

"Please. And honey."

"Two spoonfuls?"

"Right. I'll put the honey in. I like watching it drip off the spoon."

Something about her tone has caught my attention: the modulation of her voice, its unpressured directness—measured, and with a warmth I have not heard in her in months. Her eyes have softened. I caution myself not to be fooled. Yet the change in her is unmistakable.

. . . It's as if a miracle has occurred. The miracle of normalcy, of ordinary existence . . . .

It feels as if we have been living all summer inside a fable. A beautiful girl is turned into a comatose stone or a demon. She is separated from her loved ones, from language, from everything that had been hers to master. Then the spell is broken and she is awake again . . . .

After her summer of madness, Sally is able to return to school—anxious, but determined to reclaim her life. At first, she keeps her illness to herself, and enjoys the company of three close friends from her class. "Often," her father writes, "I listen to her on the phone with them, intimate, biting, gossipy—the buoyant sound of health." A few weeks into the school year, after much discussion with her parents, Sally tells her friends about her psychosis:

> *They readily accept the news. Being an alumna of the psych ward confers social status on Sally. It's a kind of credential. She has been where they have not been. It becomes their secret.*

Sally's madness resolves, and this, one might hope, would be the end of the story. But the very defining feature of manic-depressive illness is its cyclical nature, and in a postscript to his book, Greenberg indicates that Sally did have two further attacks: four years later, when she was in college, and six years after that (when her medication was discontinued). There is no "cure" for manic-depressive illness, but living with manic-depressive illness may be greatly helped by medication, by insight and understanding (in particular, by minimizing stressors like sleep loss, and being alert to the earliest signs of mania or depression), and, not least, by counseling and psychotherapy.

In its detail, depth, richness, and sheer intelligence, *Hurry Down Sunshine* will be recognized as a classic of its kind, along with the memoirs of Kay Redfield Jamison and John Custance. But what makes it unique is the fact that so much here is seen through the eyes of an extraordinarily open and sensitive parent—a father who, while never descending into sentimentality, has remarkable insight into his daughter's thoughts and feelings, and a rare power to find images or metaphors for almost unimaginable states of mind.

The question of "telling," of publishing detailed accounts of patients' lives, their vulnerabilities, their illness, is a matter of great moral delicacy, fraught with pitfalls and perils of every sort. Is Sally's struggle with psychosis not a private and personal matter, no one's business but her own (and that of her family and physicians)? Why would her father consider exposing his daughter's travails, and his family's pain, to the world? And how would Sally feel about a public disclosure of her teenage torments and exaltations?

This was not a quick or easy decision for either Sally or her father. Greenberg did not grab a pen and start writing during his daughter's psychosis in 1996—he waited, he pondered, he let the experience sink deep into him. He had long, searching discussions with Sally, and only more than a decade later did he feel that he might have the balance, the perspective, the tone that *Hurry Down Sunshine* would need. Sally, too, had come to feel this, and urged him not only to write her story, but to use

her real name, without camouflage. It was a courageous decision, given the stigma and misunderstanding that still surround
mental illness of any kind.

It is a stigma that affects many, for manic-depressive illness occurs in all cultures, and affects at least one person in a
hundred—there are, at any time, millions of people, some even
younger than Sally, who may have to face what she did. Lucid,
realistic, compassionate, illuminating, *Hurry Down Sunshine* may
provide a sort of guide for those who have to negotiate the dark
regions of the soul—a guide, too, for their families and friends,
for all those who want to understand what their loved ones are
going through. Perhaps, too, it will remind us of what a narrow
ridge of normality we all inhabit, with the abysses of mania and
depression yawning to either side.

Contagious Cancer: The Evolution of a Killer

David Quammen

From *Harper's*

DURING THE EARLY months of 1996, not long before Easter, an amateur wildlife photographer named Christo Baars made his way to the Australian island-state of Tasmania, where he set up camp in an old airport shack within the boundaries of Mount William National Park. Baars's purpose, as on previous visits, was to photograph Tasmanian devils, piglet-size marsupials unique to the island's temperate forests and moors. Because devils are nocturnal, Baars equipped his blind with a cot, a couple of car batteries, and several strong spotlights. For bait he used road-kill kangaroos. Then he settled in to wait.

The devil, known to science as *Sarcophilus harrisii*, lives mostly by scavenging and sometimes by predation. It will eat, in addition to kangaroo meat, chickens, fish, frogs, kelp maggots, lambs, rats, snakes, wallabies, and the occasional rubber boot. It can consume nearly half its own body weight in under an hour, and yet—with its black fur and its trundling gait—it looks like an underfed bear cub. Fossil evidence shows that devils inhabited all of Australia until about 500 years ago, when competition with dingoes and other factors caused them to die out everywhere but in Tasmania, which dingoes had yet to colonize. More recently, Tasmanian stockmen and farmers have persecuted devils with the same ferocity directed elsewhere at wolves and coyotes. The devils' reproductive rate, opportunistic habits, and tolerance for human proximity, however, have allowed localized populations to persist or recover, and at the time of Baars's 1996 visit, their total number was probably around 150,000.

On his earlier visits, Baars had seen at least ten devils every night, and they were quick to adjust to his presence. They would walk into his blind, into his tent, into his kitchen, and he could recognize returning individuals by the distinctively shaped white patches on their chests. This trip was different. On the first night, his bait failed to attract a single devil, and the second night was only a little better. He thought at first that maybe the stockmen and farmers had finally succeeded in wiping them out. Then he spotted a devil with a weird facial lump. It was an ugly mass, rounded and bulging, like a huge boil, or a tumor. Baars took photographs. More devils wandered in, at least one of them with a similar growth, and Baars took more pictures. This was no longer wildlife photography of the picturesque sort; it was, or anyway soon would become, forensic documentation.

Back in Hobart, Tasmania's capital, Baars showed his pictures to Nick Mooney, a veteran officer of Tasmania's Parks and Wildlife Service who has dealt with the devil and its enemies for decades. Mooney had never seen anything like this. The lumps looked tumorous, yes—but what sort of tumor? Mooney consulted a pathologist, who suggested that the devils might be afflicted with lymphosarcoma, a kind of lymphatic cancer, maybe caused by a virus passed to the devils from feral cats. Such a virus might also be passed from devil to devil, triggering cancer in each.

More evidence of contagion began to accumulate. Three years after Baars shot his photographs, a biologist named Menna Jones took note of a single tumor-bearing animal, something she had not seen before. Then, in 2001, at her study site along Tasmania's eastern coast, her traps yielded three more devils with ulcerated tumors. That really got her attention. She euthanized the animals and brought them to a lab, where they became the first victims to be autopsied by a veterinary pathologist. The "tumors" (until then the term had been only a guess or a metaphor) did seem to be cancerous malignancies, but not of the sort expected from a lymphosarcoma- triggering virus. This peculiarity raised more questions than it answered. Tasmanian devils in captivity were known to be quite susceptible to cancer, at least in some circumstances, possibly involving exposure to carcinogens. But the idea that the cancer itself was contagious seemed beyond the realm of possibility. And yet, during the following year, Menna Jones charted the spread of the problem across northern Tasmania. Nick Mooney, meanwhile, had done some further trapping himself. At a site in the northern midlands, he captured twenty-three devils, seven of which had horrible tumors. Shocked and puzzled, he remembered the Baars photos from years earlier.

Further trapping (more than a hundred animals, of which 15 percent were infected) showed Mooney what Jones had also seen: that the tumors were consistently localized on faces, filling eye sockets, distending cheeks, making it difficult for the animals to see or to eat. Why faces? Maybe because devils suffer many facial and mouth injuries—from chewing on brittle bones, from fighting with one another over food and breeding rights, from the rough interactions between male and female when they mate. The bigger tumors were crumbly, like feta cheese. Could it be that tumor cells, broken off one animal, fell into the wounds of another, took hold there, and grew? This prospect seemed outlandish, but the evidence was leading inexorably to a strange and frightening new hypothesis: the cancer itself had somehow become contagious.

Under ordinary circumstances, cancer is an individuated phenomenon. Its onset is determined partly by genetics, partly by environment, partly by entropy, partly by the remorseless tick-tock of time, and (almost) never by the transmission of some tumorous essence. It arises from within (usually) rather than being imposed from without. It pinpoints single victims (usually) rather than spreading through populations. Cancer might be triggered by a carcinogenic chemical, but it isn't itself poisoning. It might be triggered by a virus, but it isn't fundamentally viral. Cancer differs also from heart disease and cirrhosis and the other lethal forms of physiological breakdown; uncontrolled cell reproduction, not organ dilapidation, is the problem.

Such uncontrolled reproduction begins when a single cell accumulates enough mutations to activate certain growth-promoting genes (scientists call them oncogenes) and to inactivate certain protections (tumor suppressor genes) that are built into the genetic program of every animal and plant. The cell ignores instructions to limit its self-replication, and soon it becomes many cells, all of them similarly demented, all bent on self-replication, all heedless of duty and proportion and the larger weal of the organism. That first cell is (almost always) a cell of the victim's own body. So cancer is reinvented from scratch on a case-by-case basis, and this individuation, this personalization, may be one of the reasons that it seems so frightening and solitary. But what makes it even more solitary for its victims is the idea, secretly comforting to others, that cancer is never contagious. That idea is axiomatic, at least in the popular consciousness. *Cancer is not an infectious disease.* And the axiom is (usually) correct. But there are exceptions. Those exceptions point toward a broader reality that scientists have begun to explore: Cancers, like species, evolve. And one way they can evolve is toward the capacity to be transmitted between individuals.

Devil tumor isn't the only form of cancer ever to achieve such a feat. Other cases have occurred and are still occurring. The most notable is Canine Transmissible Venereal Tumor (CTVT), also called Sticker's sarcoma, a sexually transmitted malignancy in dogs. Again, this is not merely an infectious virus that tends to induce cancer. The tumor cells themselves are transmitted during sexual contact. CTVT is widespread (though not common) and has been claiming dogs around the world at least since a Russian veterinarian named M. A. Novinsky first noted it in 1876. The distinctively altered chromosome patterns shared by the cells of CTVT show the cancer's lineal continuity, its identity across space and through time. Tumor cells in Dog B, Dog C, Dog D, and Dog Z are more closely related to one another than those cells are to the dogs they respectively inhabit. In other words, CTVT can be conceptualized as a single creature, a parasite (and not a *species* of parasite, but an *individual*), which has managed to spread itself out among millions of different dogs. Research by molecular geneticists suggests the tumor originated in a wolf, or maybe an East Asian dog, somewhere between 200 and 2,500 years ago, which means that CTVT is probably the oldest continuous lineage of mammal cells presently living on Earth. The dogs may be young, but the tumor is ancient.

Unlike devil tumor—now known as Devil Facial Tumor Disease, or DFTD—CTVT is generally not fatal. It can be cured with veterinary surgery or chemotherapy. In many cases, even without treatment, the dog's immune system eventually recognizes the CTVT as alien, attacks it, and clears it away, just as our own immune systems eventually rid us of warts.

The case of the Syrian hamster is more complicated. This tumor arose around 1960, when researchers at the National Cancer Institute, in Bethesda, Maryland, performed an experiment in which they harvested a naturally occurring sarcoma from one hamster and injected those cells (as cancer scientists often do) into healthy animals. When the injected hamsters developed malignancies, more cells were harvested. Each such inoculation-

and-harvest cycle is called a passage. The experiment involved a dozen such passages, and over time the tumor began to change. It had evolved. The later generations, unlike the first, represented a sort of super tumor, capable of getting from hamster to hamster without benefit of a needle. The researchers caged ten healthy hamsters together with ten cancerous hamsters and found that nine of the healthy animals acquired tumors through social contact. The hamster tumor had leapt between animals—or anyway, it had been smeared, spat, bitten, and dribbled between them. (The tenth hamster got cannibalized before it could sicken.) In a related experiment, the tumor even passed between two hamsters separated by a wire screen. The scientists had in effect created a laboratory precursor of what would eventually afflict Tasmanian devils in the wild: a Frankenstein malignancy, a leaping tumor, which could conceivably kill off not just individuals but an entire species.

Early last summer I went to Tasmania, where I met Menna Jones for an excursion to the Forestier Peninsula, a long hook of land that juts southeastward into the Tasman Sea. Jones supervises an experimental trapping program aimed at ridding the peninsula of tumor disease or, at least, determining whether that goal is achievable. The Forestier is a good place for such trials because the peninsula (and its lower extension, a second lobe called the Tasman Peninsula) is connected to the rest of Tasmania by only a narrow neck—just a two-lane bridge across a canal. If the disease could be eradicated from the entire peninsula, by removing all sick animals and leaving the healthy ones, Forestier and Tasman might be protected from re-infection by a devil-proof barrier across the bridge; and if that worked, the protected population could rebound quickly. The Forestier Peninsula, full of good habitat, might become a vital refuge for the species. Those measures might even validate a method—defense by tourniquet—that could be used on some of Tasmania's other peninsular arms.

Jones, who is a brisk, cordial woman with a mane of brown hair, picked me up in an official state Land Cruiser, and as she drove she described the effects seen so far. Her field people had culled more than a hundred devils within the past four months, she said, and though the size of the Forestier population seemed to be holding steady, the demographics had changed. Mature adults, the four- and five-year-olds, were being lost, and so three-year-olds, adolescents, were accounting for most of the parent-hood. The biting associated with breeding brings fatal disease, and the disease kills fast—sex equals death, a bad equation for any species. "We think extinction is a possibility within twenty-five years," Jones said.

We crossed the little bridge onto the peninsula and, after a short drive through rolling hills of eucalyptus forest, rendez-voused with the trapping crew. The chief trapper was a young woman named Chrissy Pukk, Estonian by descent, Aussie by man-ner, wearing a pair of blue coveralls, a dangling surgical mask, and a leather bush hat. She had been trapping devils here for three years. Jones and I tagged along as Pukk and two volunteers worked a line of forty traps placed throughout the forest. The catch rate was high, and most of the captured devils had been caught previously and injected with small electronic inserts for identification. These devils came in on a regular basis, as if the traps were soup kitchens, and Pukk recognized many of them on sight. She and only she handled the animals, cooing to them calmingly while she took their measurements, checked their body condition, and, most crucially, examined their faces for injuries and signs of tumor. One devil, a robust male Pukk called Captain Bligh, showed wounds from a recent mating session: broken teeth, a torn nose, a half-healed cut below his jaw, and a suppurating pink hole on the top of his snout, deep enough that it might have been made by a melon scoop. But he seemed to be clean of tumor's just a brawler," Pukk said. She released him, and he skittered off into the brush.

"You see a lot of old friends come and go," Pukk told me as she examined another animal. For instance, there was one she had caught the day before, a male called Noddy. She had last trapped him less than a week earlier, noted inflamed whisker roots, and released him; but in the brief passage of days, those inflammations had become tumors, and now Noddy was awaiting his fate in a holding trap.

Colette Harmsen, a veterinarian who had made the long drive south from Tasmania's Animal Health Laboratory at Mount Pleasant, was there to euthanize and autopsy any animal Pukk found unfit for release. She wore her black hair cut short, her jeans torn at the knee, a lacey black dress over the jeans, a black T-shirt reading save tassie's forests over the dress, and, over it all, a pale blue disposable surgical smock. She was waiting at her pickup truck along with her pit bull, Lily, and her pet rat, CC, when Pukk arrived to deliver the unfortunate Noddy. Pukk and her crew returned to the trap line, Menna Jones went back to Hobart, and I stayed to watch Harmsen work. I had never seen anyone cut open a Tasmanian devil.

Her working slab was the tailgate of her pickup, spread with a clean burlap sack; her scalpels, syringes, and other tools came from a portable kit. First she anesthetized Noddy with gas. Then, after drawing blood samples from deep in his heart, she injected him with something called Lethabarb, which killed him. She measured his carcass, inspected his face, and then sliced an olive-size lump off his right cheek just below the eye. She showed me the lump's interior: a pea-size core of pale tissue surrounded by normal pink flesh. She put a chunk of it into a vial; that would go to a lab up at Mount Pleasant, she said, to be grown for chromosome typing. From the left side of the face, among the whiskers, Harmsen cut another tumor. Noddy lay limp on the burlap, both cheeks sliced away, like a halibut. When she slit open his belly and found an abundance of healthy yellow fat, she sighed. "He was in good condition." The disease hadn't progressed far. There was no sign of metastasis. But the protocols of the trapping program on Forestier don't include therapeutic surgery and chemo. Harmsen put a bit of Noddy's liver, a bit of his spleen, and a bit of his kidney into formalin. Those samples, too, would go back to Mount Pleasant for analysis. She wrapped the rest of Noddy in his burlap shroud, put him in a plastic garbage bag, and sealed that with tape. He would be incinerated. Then she cleaned up, fastidiously, to eliminate the chance that tumor cells might pass from her tailgate or her tools to another animal.

The phenomenon of transmissible tumors isn't confined to canines, Tasmanian devils, and Syrian hamsters. There have been human cases, too. Forty years ago a team of physicians led by Edward F. Scanlon reported, in the journal *Cancer*, that they had "decided to transplant small pieces of tumor from a cancer patient into a healthy donor, on a well informed volunteer basis, in the hope of gaining a little better understanding of cancer immunity," which they thought might help in treating the patient. The patient was a fifty-year-old woman with advanced melanoma; the "donor" was her healthy eighty-year-old mother, who had agreed to receive a bit of the tumor by surgical transplant. One day after the transplant procedure, the daughter died suddenly from a perforated bowel. Scanlon's report neglects to explain why the experiment wasn't promptly terminated—why they didn't dive back in surgically to undo what had been done to the mother. Instead, three weeks were allowed to pass, at which point the mother had developed a tumor indistinguishable from her daughter's. Now it was too late for surgery. This cancer moved fast. It metastasized, and the mother died about fifteen months later, with tumors in her lungs, ribs, lymph nodes, and diaphragm.

The case of the daughter–mother transplant and the case of the Syrian hamsters have one common element: the original sources of the tumor and the recipients were genetically very similar. If the genome of one individual closely resembles the genome of another (as children resemble their parents, and as inbred animals resemble one another), the immune system of a recipient may not detect the foreignness of transplanted cells. The hamsters were highly inbred (intentionally, for experimental control) and therefore not very individuated from one another as far as their immune systems could discern. The mother and daughter were also genetically similar—as similar as two people can be without being identical twins. Lack of normal immune response, because of such closeness, goes some way toward explaining why those tumors survived transference between individuals.

Low immune response also figures in two other situations in which tumor transmission is known to occur: pregnancy and organ transplant. A mother sometimes passes cancer cells to her fetus in the womb. And a transplanted organ sometimes carries tiny tumors into the recipient, vitiating the benefits of receiving a life-saving liver or kidney from someone else. Cases of both kinds are very rare, and they involve some inherent or arranged compatibility between the original victim of the tumor and the secondary victim, plus an immune system that is either compromised (by immuno-suppressive drugs, in the organ recipient) or immature (in the fetus).

Other cases are less easily explained. In 1986, two researchers from the National Institutes of Health reported that a laboratory worker, a healthy nineteen-year-old woman, had accidentally jabbed herself with a syringe carrying colon-cancer cells; a colonic tumor grew in her hand, but she was rescued by surgery. More recently, a fifty-three-year-old surgeon cut his left palm while removing a malignancy from a patient's abdomen, and five months later he found himself with a palm tumor, one that genetically matched the patient's tumor. His immune system responded, creating an inflammation around the tumor, but the response was insufficient and the tumor kept growing. Why? How? It wasn't supposed to be able to do that. Again, though, surgery delivered a full cure. And then there's Henri Vadon. He was a medical student in the 1920s who poked his left hand with a syringe after drawing liquid from the mastectomy wound of a woman being treated for breast cancer. Vadon, too, developed a hand tumor. Three years later, he died of metastasized cancer because neither the surgical techniques of his era nor his own immune system could save him.

The tumor that I had watched Colette Harmsen harvest from Noddy's face would be examined at the Mount Pleasant labs by Anne-Maree Pearse and her assistant Kate Swift. Pearse is a former parasitologist, now working in cell biology, and she has a special interest in the genetics of Devil Facial Tumor Disease. She and Swift were the researchers who, in 2006, published a dramatic report in the British journal *Nature* that, with eight paragraphs of text and a single photographic image, had answered the lingering question about whether DFTD is a genuinely transmissible cancer.

Pearse came out of retirement (she had turned to running a flower farm) in response to the scientific conundrum of DFTD. A back injury has forced the use of a cane on her, but she is vigorous when describing her research. Although she was originally trained as an entomologist, her work with fleas drew her into the world of parasitology, and from there it was just a few more steps into oncology and the study of lymphomas among the devil and its close marsupial relatives. "Somehow my whole life was preparing me for this," she said when I visited her lab at Mount Pleasant. She added, almost appreciatively: "This disease." Pearse tends to think, as she put it, "outside the square"—a useful trait in the case of DFTD, she said, because the disease isn't behaving like anything heretofore known. "It's a parasitic cancer," she told me. "The devil's the host."

For the 2006 study, Pearse and Swift examined chromosome structure in tumor cells from eleven different devils. They found that the tumor chromosomes were abnormal (misshapen, some missing, some added) compared with those from healthy devil cells, but that the tumor chromosomes, from one cell or another, from one tumor or another, were abnormal in *all the same ways*.

You could see that comparison graphically in the photo in *Nature*: fourteen nice sausages matched against thirteen variously mangled ones. Those thirteen chromosomes, wrote Pearse and Swift, had undergone "a complex rearrangement that is identical for every animal studied." The mangling was unmistakable evidence. It appeared in each tumor, but not elsewhere in each animal. "In light of this remarkable finding and of the known fighting behavior of the devils," Pearse and Swift wrote, "we propose that the disease is transmitted by allograft"—tissue transplant—"whereby an infectious cell line is passed directly between the animals through bites they inflict on one another."

Pearse and Swift had proved that DFTD is a highly infectious form of cancer, its transmission made possible by, among other factors, the habit of mutual face-biting. When I visited Menna Jones, she expressed the same idea: "It's a piece of devil tissue that behaves like a parasite." Jones was using the word "parasite" in its strict biological sense, meaning: any organism that lives on or within another kind of organism, extracting benefit for itself and causing harm to the other. The first rule of a successful parasite is, Don't kill your host—or at least, Don't kill one host until you've had time to leap aboard another. DFTD, passing quickly from devil to devil, killing them all but not quite so quickly, follows that rule.

How does any parasite, whether it is a species or merely a tumor, acquire the attributes and tactics necessary for survival, reproduction, and continuing success? The answer is simple but not obvious: evolution.

Cancer and evolution have traditionally been considered separately by different scientists with different interests using different methods. You could graduate from medical school, you could follow that with a Ph.D. in cell biology or molecular genetics, you could become a respected oncologist or a well-funded cancer researcher, without ever having read Darwin. You could do it, in fact, without having studied much evolutionary biology at all. Many cell and molecular biologists tended even to scorn evolutionary biology as a "merely descriptive" enterprise, lacking the rigor, quantifiability, and explanatory power of their disciplines. There were exceptions to this disconnect, cancer scientists who even during the early days thought in evolutionary terms, but those scientists had little influence.

In recent decades, however, the situation has changed, as molecular genetics and evolutionary biology have converged on some shared questions. One signal act of synthesis occurred in 1976 when a leukemia researcher named Peter Nowell published a theoretical paper in *Science* titled "The Clonal Evolution of Tumor Cell Populations." Nowell proposed what was then a novel idea: that the biological events occurring when cells progress from normal to pre-cancerous to cancerous represent a form of evolution by natural selection. As with the evolution of species, he suggested, the evolution of malignant tumors requires two conditions: genetic diversity among the individuals of a population and competition among those individuals for limited resources. Genetic diversity within one mass of pre-cancerous cells comes from mutations—copying errors and other forms of change—that yield variants as the cells reproduce. That is, in the very act of replicating themselves (sometimes inaccurately), the cells diversify into a population encompassing some small genetic differences between one cell and another. Each variant cell then replicates itself true to type, constituting a clonal lineage (a lineage of accurate copies), until the next mutation creates a new variant. The fittest variants survive and proliferate. By this means, the genetic character of the cell population gradually changes, and with such change comes adaptation, a better fit to environmental circumstances. What constitutes "the fittest" among clonal lineages within a pre-cancerous growth? Those that can reproduce fastest. Those that can resist chemotherapy. Those that can metastasize and therefore escape the surgeon's knife.

Nowell's hypothesis about tumor evolution became widely known and accepted within certain circles of cancer research.

(Among other researchers, it wasn't adamantly disputed but merely ignored.) Those circles have more recently produced a lot of rich theorizing, and a smaller amount of empirical work, supporting Nowell and carrying his idea forward. A culmination of sorts occurred in 2000, when the cancer geneticist Robert Weinberg, discoverer of the first human oncogene and the first tumor suppressor gene, published a concise paper titled "The Hallmarks of Cancer." Weinberg and his coauthor, Doug las Hanahan, described six "acquired capabilities," such as endless self-replication, the ignoring of antigrowth signals, the invasion of neighboring tissues, and the refusal to die, that collectively characterize cancer cells. How are those capabilities acquired? By mutations and other genetic changes, giving cells with one such trait or another competitive advantage over normal cells. Hanahan and Weinberg added that "tumor development proceeds via a process formally analogous to Darwinian evolution." With this cautious phrasing, they gave authoritative endorsement to the idea that Peter Nowell had proposed: Cancers, like species, evolve.

In 1998 a young researcher named Carlo Maley began looking for a way to study the evolution of cancer. Educated at Oxford and MIT as an evolutionary biologist and a computer modeler, Maley had no training in medicine and not much in molecular biology. During a postgraduate fellowship, though, he became interested in infectious disease. He figured that if evolution was cool, then coevolution—wherein both parasite and host are evolving—would be doubly cool. Then he stumbled across a description of cancer as an evolving disease. He read that Sir Walter Bodmer, a British geneticist and the former director of the Imperial Cancer Research Fund, had urged his cancer-research colleagues to "think evolution, evolution, evolution" when they considered tumor cells. Maley typed "evolution and cancer" into a search engine for the scientific literature, which turned up very little. He did learn of Nowell's hypothesis, but that was just theory. He was groping. He had done plenty of theoretical modeling, but for this task he needed the desperate realities, and the data, of clinical oncology.

And then, at a workshop in Seattle, Maley met Brian Reid, an experienced cancer researcher studying something called Barrett's esophagus, a pre-cancerous condition of the lower throat. They hit it off. Reid had the right clinical situation but wasn't deeply versed in evolutionary biology; Maley had the right background. They agreed to collaborate.

Reid and his colleagues possessed sixteen years of continuous data on Barrett's patients and a tissue bank going back to 1989. They knew which patients had developed esophageal cancer and which hadn't, and they could match those outcomes against what they had seen in cell cultures and genetic work from earlier in the patients' history. So they could ask evolutionary questions that were answerable from patterns in the data. The most basic question was: Did tumors become malignant through evolution by natural selection? The other big question was: Can doctors predict which pre-cancerous growths will turn malignant? Maley and Reid, along with additional collaborators, found that case histories of Barrett's esophagus tend to confirm Nowell's hypothesis. Cancerous tumors, like species, *do* evolve. And from the Barrett's data, predictions can be made. The higher the diversity of different cell variants within a pre-cancerous growth, the greater the likelihood that the growth will progress to malignancy. Why? Because of the basic Darwinian mechanism. Genetic diversity plus competitive struggle eliminates unfit individuals and leaves the well-adapted to reproduce.

Maley and Reid have more recently taken such thinking one step beyond evolution—into ecology. Along with Lauren M. F. Merlo (as first author) and John W. Pepper, they published a provocative paper titled "Cancer as an Evolutionary and Ecological Process," in which they discussed not just tumor evolution but also the ecological factors that form evolution's context, such as predation, parasitism, competition, dispersal, and colonization. Dispersal is travel by venturesome individuals, which in some cases allows species to colonize new habitats. Merlo, Maley, and their colleagues noted three ways in which the concept of dispersal is applicable to cancer: small-scale cell movement within a tumor (not very important), invasion of neighboring tissues (important), and metastasis (fateful).

Reading that, I remembered Devil Facial Tumor Disease and wondered whether there might not be a fourth way: transmissibility. An infectious cancer is a successful disperser. It colonizes new habitat. DFTD seems to be dispersing and colonizing, much as pigeons disperse across oceans, colonizing new islands. This wasn't just evolution; it was evolutionary ecology.

I called one of the paper's coauthors, John W. Pepper, an evolutionary biologist at the University of Arizona, and asked whether I was stretching the notion too far. No, he said, you're not. If he could revise that paper again, Pepper told me, he would insert the idea that tumors evolve toward transmissibility.

Eight hundred million years ago there was no such thing as cancer. Virtually all living creatures were single-celled organisms, and the rule was *Every cell for itself!* Uncontrolled, undifferentiated cell growth wasn't abnormal. It was the program of all life on Earth.

Then, around 700 million years ago, things changed. Paleontologists call this event the Cambrian explosion. Complex multicellular animals, metazoans, appeared. And not just meta-*zoans* but meta*phytes,* too—that is, multicellular plants. How did it happen? Very gradually, as single-cell creatures resembling bacteria or algae began to aggregate into colonial units and discover, by trial and error, how they could benefit from division of labor and specialization of shape and function. To enjoy those benefits, they had to set aside the old rule of absolute selfishness. They had to cooperate. They couldn't cheat against the interests of the collective entity. (Or anyway they *shouldn't* cheat, not very often; otherwise the benefits of collectivity wouldn't accrue.) Cooperation was a winning formula. Primitive multicellular creatures, roughly along the lines of jellyfish or sponges or slime molds, began to succeed, to grow, to occupy space, and to claim resources in ways that loner cells couldn't. You can see their imprints in the Burgess Shale: weird things like sci-fi vermin, pre-vertebrate, pre-insect, that seem to have been built out of bubble wrap and old Slinkys. They succeeded for a while, then gave way to still better designs. Multicellularity offered wide possibilities.

But uncontrolled cell replication didn't disappear entirely. Sometimes a single atavistic cell would ignore the collective imperative; it would revert to the old habit—proliferating wildly, disregarding all signals to stop. It would swell into a big, greedy lump of its own kind, and in so doing disrupt one or more of the necessary collective functions. That was cancer.

The risk of runaway cell replication remained a factor in the evolutionary process, even as multicellular creatures increased vastly in complexity, diversity, size, and dominance on our planet. And species responded to that risk just as they responded, incrementally and over long periods of time, to other such risks as predation or parasitism: by acquiring defenses. One such defense is the amazing ability of living cells to repair mutated DNA, putting the cell program back together properly after a mishap during cell replication. Another defense is *apoptosis,* a form of programming that tells a cell not to live forever. Another is cellular senescence, during which a cell continues to live but no longer is capable of replicating. Another is the distinction between stem cells and differentiated cells, which limits the number of cells responsible for cell-replacement activity and thereby reduces the risk of accumulated mutations. Another is the requirement for biochemical growth signals before a cell can begin to proliferate. Many of these defenses are controlled by tumor-suppressor genes, such as the one that produces a protein that prevents cells from replicating damaged DNA. Nobody knows just how many anti-cancer defenses exist within a given species (we humans seem to have more than mice do, and possibly not so many as whales), but we do know that they make our continuing lives possible.

Tumors, in the course of their own evolution from one normal cell to a cancerous malignancy, circumvent these natural defenses. They may also change in response to externally imposed defenses, such as surgery, chemotherapy, and radiation. The fittest cells, in Darwinian terms, are those that reproduce themselves most quickly and aggressively, resisting all signals to desist and all attempts to kill them. The victim (that is, the human or the Tasmanian devil or the Syrian hamster) suffers the consequences, having become the arena for an evolutionary struggle at a scale far different from that of its own struggle to survive. But the principles of the struggle are the same at each scale.

This process, whereby cells mutate, reproduce, and proliferate differentially within a body, is called somatic evolution. It stands as a counterpoint to organismic evolution (progressive changes at the scale of whole bodies within a population), and the opportunities for it to proceed are abundant. According to one count, at least 291 genes in the human body contribute, when damaged by mutation, toward somatic evolution.

Mutations occur when something goes wrong during cell replication. A cell replicates by copying its DNA (sometimes inaccurately), sorting the DNA into two identical parcels of chromosomes, then splitting into two new cells, each with its own chromosomes. This process is called mitosis. The goal is not to generate an ever-higher number of cells during a creature's adult lifetime but simply to replace old cells with new ones. Mitosis counterbalanced with apoptosis, cell death, should provide a constant supply. But each time a mitotic division occurs, there is some very small chance of mutation. And the many small chances add up. A human body contains about 30 trillion cells. The number of cell divisions that occur in a lifetime is far larger: 10,000 trillion. A disproportionately large share of those divisions occurs in epithelial cells, which serve as boundary layers or linings, such as the skin and the interior surface of the colon. That's why skin cancer and colon cancer are relatively common—more cell turnover, more chance of mutation and evolution.

How many mutations does it take for a malignancy to occur? Estimates range from three to twelve, in humans, depending on the form of cancer. Five or six is considered an operational average for purposes of discussion. Here's some good news: For a cell to acquire those five or six changes, at the usual rate of mutation, is highly, highly, highly unlikely. The odds are great against quintuple mutation in any given cell, making cancer seem impossible within a human lifespan. One form of mutation, however, can vastly increase the later rate of mutation, which gives the precancerous cells many more chances to become malignant.

In the United States, about 40 percent of us will eventually get cancer bad enough to be diagnosed. And autopsies suggest that virtually all of us will be nurturing incipient thyroid cancer by the time we die. Among octogenarian and nonagenarian men, 80 percent carry prostate cancer when they go. Cancer is terrible, cancer is dramatic, but cancer isn't rare. In fact, it's nearly universal.

The biological mystery of how the Tasmanian devil's rogue tumor manages to establish itself in one animal after another is still unsolved. But a good hypothesis has been offered by an immunologist named Greg Woods at the University of Tasmania. Woods and his group studied immune reactions in *Sarcophilus harrisii*, which seem generally to be normal against ordinary sorts of infection. Against DFTD cells, though, no such reaction occurs. "The tumor is just not *seen* by the immune system, because it just looks too similar," Woods told me when I stopped by his lab. The devils have low genetic diversity, probably because they inhabit a small island, they colonized it originally by way of just a few founders, and they have passed through some tight population bottlenecks in the centuries since. They're not quite so alike one another as a bunch of inbred hamsters, but they're too alike for their own good in the current sad, anomalous circumstances. Their immune systems don't reject the tumor cells because, Woods suspects, in each animal the critical MHC genes (the major histocompatibility complex, which produces proteins crucial to immunological policing) are all virtually identical, and the devils' police cells can't distinguish "him" from "me."

Most of the DFTD team are, like Greg Woods and Anne-Maree Pearse, located in Hobart or Launceston. Most of the animals aren't. So, two days after the autopsy on Noddy, I drove back to the Forestier Peninsula for another round of trapping with Chrissy Pukk and her crew. It wasn't that I expected to learn any new angles on the science. I just wanted to see more Tasmanian devils.

This time, Pukk issued me my own pair of blue coveralls. As we set off along the trap line, she exuded the contentment of a joyously crude tomboy enjoying the best job in the world: trapping devils for the good of the species. The only downside was the necessity of issuing a death sentence to any animal with a trace of tumor. "You get attached to the individuals," she admitted. "But you've got to remember all the other individuals you can save if you take that animal out early on."

Wouldn't this be less difficult emotionally, I asked her, if you gave them *numbers* instead of names? She answered the question—saying she couldn't do her work properly if she wasn't emotionally invested, plus which, names were easier to remember—and then she continued to answer it throughout the day. These creatures, they all have their memorable eccentricities, their little histories, she explained. Some she could recognize almost by smell. You couldn't do *that* with numbers.

There were forty traps again today, and about a dozen trapped devils to process, all recaptures, previously tagged and named. Trap by trap, animal by animal, Pukk worked through the measurements and the facial exams, handling each devil firmly but with a steady touch that provoked no devilish squirming: Captain Bligh (looking glum, or maybe a little embarrassed at having been caught again so soon), Hipster, Isabel, Masikus (Estonian for "strawberry"), Miss Buzzy Bum (her rump had been full of burrs), Rudolph (thus called for a nose that had been rubbed raw), Sandman, Skipper, and many others. They may have been virtually indistinguishable in the terms by which immune systems operate, but Chrissy Pukk knew each devil at a glance.

Rudolph's condition gave her pause. He was a two-year-old, nicely grown since she had first trapped him, his red nose healed . . . but there was something on the edge of his right eye. A pink growth, no bigger than a caper. "Oh shit," she said. Tumor? Or maybe it was just a little wound, puffy and raw. She looked closely. She peered into his mouth. She palpated lymph nodes at the base of his jaw. The volunteers and I waited in silence. Evolution had shaped Rudolph for survival, and evolution might take him away. It was all evolution: the yin of struggle and death, the yang of adaptation, DFTD versus *Sarcophilus harrisii*. The leaping tumor, well adapted for fast replication and transmissibility, has its own formidable impulse to survive. And no one could know at this point, not even Chrissy, whether it had already leapt into Rudolph.

"Okay," she said, sounding almost sure of her judgment, "I'm gonna give him the all clear." She released him and he ran.

At latest report, Devil Facial Tumor Disease has spread across 60 percent of Tasmania's land surface, and in some areas, especially where it got its earliest start, the devil population seems to have declined by as much as 90 percent. In November, the Tasmanian government classified the devil as "endangered." DFTD specialists differ strongly on how such a crisis should be met. One view is that suppressing the disease— trapping and euthanizing as many infected animals as possible and then establishing barriers, as on the Forestier Peninsula—is the best strategy. Another view is that the species, virtually doomed on mainland Tasmania, can better be saved by transplanting disease-free devils to a small offshore island. Still another view, maybe the boldest and most risky, is that doing nothing— allowing the disease to spread unchecked—might yield a small remnant population of survivors, with natural immunity to DFTD, who could repopulate Tasmania.

Weeks after my last outing with the trappers, back in the Northern Hemisphere and wanting a broader perspective—not just on the fate of the devils but on the evolution of cancer—I met Robert Weinberg at a stem-cell conference in Big Sky, Montana. Because it was a Sunday, with the first session not yet convened, and because he is a genial man, Weinberg gave me a two-hour tutorial in a boardroom of the ski lodge, fortifying some points by flipping through his own four-pound textbook, *The Biology of Cancer,* a copy of which I had lugged to our meeting like a student. He was incognito in a plaid Woolrich shirt. He'd be called on that evening to deliver the keynote address, but never mind, he was prepared.

"Infectious cancer is really an aberration," Weinberg told me, affirming what Greg Woods had said. "It's so bizarre. It has happened only rarely." Maybe it's possible only in cases where there's close physical contact between susceptible tissues. "That, right away, limits it to venereal tumors, or tumors that can be transmitted by biting." Weinberg knew that I'd walked in with a head full of Tasmanian devils.

Does this mean that cancer cells are harder to transmit than, say, virus particles? "Much," he said. "Cells are very *effete.* Very susceptible to dying in the outside world." They dry out, they wither, they don't remain viable when they're naked and alone. Bacteria can form spores. Viruses in their capsules can lie dormant. But cells from a metazoan? No. They're not packaged for transit.

And that's only one of two major constraints, Weinberg said. The second is that if cancer cells *do* pass from one body to another, they are instantly recognized as foreign and eliminated by the immune system. Each cell of any sort bears on its exterior a set of protuberant proteins that declare its identity; they might be thought of as its travel papers. These proteins are called antigens and are produced uniquely in each individual by the MHC (major histocompatibility complex) genes. If the travel papers of a cell are unacceptable (because the cell is an invader from some other body), the T cells (one type of immunological police cell) will attack and obliterate it. If the invader cell shows no papers at all, another kind of police cell (called NK cells) will bust it. Only if the antigens on the cell surface have been "downregulated" discreetly but not eliminated altogether can a foreign cell elude the immune system of a host. That's what Canine Transmissible Venereal Tumor seems to have done: downregulated its antigens. It shows fake travel papers—blurry, faded, but just good enough to get by.

Nice trick! How did CTVT do that? Although nobody knows exactly, the best hypothesis is evolution by natural selection—or by some process "formally analogous" to it.

Weinberg went on to explain that the process is a little more complicated than classic Darwinian selection. Darwin's version works by selection among genetic variations that differentiate one organism from another, and in sexually reproducing species those variations are heritable. But evolution in tumor lineages occurs by that sort of selection plus another sort—selection among *epigenetic* modifications of DNA. Epigenetic means outside the line of genetic inheritance: acquired by experience, by accident, by circumstance. Such secondary chemical changes to the molecule affect behavior, affect shape, and pass from one cell to another but do *not,* contrary to the analogy, pass from parent to offspring in sexual reproduction. These changes are peeled away in the process of meiosis (the formation of sperm and egg cells for sexual reproduction) but preserved in mitosis (the process of simple cell replication in the body). So cancerous cell reproduction brings such changes forward into the new cells, along with the fundamental genetic changes.

Does that mean tumors don't evolve? Certainly not. They do. "It's still Darwin," Weinberg said. "It's Darwin revised."

DNA Pollution May Be Spawning Killer Microbes

Jessica Snyder Sachs

from *Discover*

ROGUE GENETIC SNIPPETS spread antibiotic resistance all over the environment.

On a bright winter morning high in the Colorado Rockies, a slight young woman in oversize hip boots sidles up to a gap of open water in the icy Cache la Poudre River. Heather Storteboom, a 25-year-old graduate student at nearby Colorado State University, is prospecting for clues to an invisible killer.

Storteboom snaps on a pair of latex gloves and stretches over the frozen ledge to fill a sterile plastic jug with water. Then, setting the container aside, she swings her rubber-clad legs into the stream. "Ahh, no leaks," she says, standing upright. She pulls out a clean trowel and attempts to collect some bottom sediment; in the rapid current, it takes a half dozen tries to fill the small vial she will take back to the DNA laboratory of her adviser, environmental engineer Amy Pruden. As Storteboom packs to leave, a curious hiker approaches. "What were you collecting?" he asks. "Antibiotic resistance genes," she answers.

Storteboom and Pruden are at the leading edge of an international forensic investigation into a potentially colossal new health threat: DNA pollution. Specifically, the researchers are seeking out snippets of rogue genetic material that transforms annoying bacteria into unstoppable supergerms, immune to many or all modern antibiotics. Over the past 60 years, genes for antibiotic resistance have gone from rare to commonplace in the microbes that routinely infect our bodies. The newly resistant strains have been implicated in some 90,000 potentially fatal infections a year in the United States, higher than the number of automobile and homicide deaths combined.

Among the most frightening of the emerging pathogens is invasive MRSA, or methicillin-resistant Staphylococcus aureus. Outbreaks of MRSA in public schools recently made headlines, but that is just the tip of the iceberg. Researchers estimate that invasive MRSA kills more than 18,000 Americans a year, more than AIDS, and the problem is growing rapidly. MRSA caused just 2 percent of staph infections in 1974; in the last few years, that figure has reached nearly 65 percent. Most reported staph infections stem from MRSA born and bred in our antibiotic-drenched hospitals and nursing homes. But about 15 percent now involve strains that arose in the general community.

It is not just MRSA that is causing concern; antibiotic resistance in general is spreading alarmingly. A 2003 study of the mouths of healthy kindergartners found that 97 percent harbored bacteria with genes for resistance to four out of six tested antibiotics. In all, resistant microbes made up around 15 percent of the children's oral bacteria, even though none of the children had taken antibiotics in the previous three months. Such resistance genes are rare to nonexistent in specimens of human tissue and body fluid taken 60 years ago, before the use of antibiotics became widespread.

In part, modern medicine is paying the price for its own success. "Antibiotics may be the most powerful evolutionary force seen on this planet in billions of years," says Tufts University microbiologist Stuart Levy, author of *The Antibiotic Paradox: How the Misuse of Antibiotics Destroys Their Curative Powers*. By their nature, antibiotics support the rise of any bug that can shrug off their effects, by conveniently eliminating the susceptible competition.

But the rapid rise of bacterial genes for drug resistance stems from more than lucky mutation, Levy adds. The vast majority of these genes show a complexity that could have been achieved only over millions of years. Rather than rising anew in each species, the genes spread via the microbial equivalent of sexual promiscuity. Bacteria swap genes, not only among their own kind but also between widely divergent species, Levy explains. Bacteria can even scavenge the naked DNA that spills from their dead compatriots out into the environment.

The result is a microbial arms-smuggling network with a global reach. Over the past 50 years, virtually every known kind of disease-causing bacterium has acquired genes to survive some or all of the drugs that once proved effective against it. Analysis of a strain of vancomycin-resistant enterococcus, a potentially lethal bug that has invaded many hospitals, reveals that more than one-quarter of its genome—including virtually all its antibiotic-thwarting genes—is made up of foreign DNA. One of the newest banes of U.S. medical centers, a supervirulent and multidrug-resistant strain of *Acinetobacter baumannii*, likewise appears to have picked up most of its resistance in gene swaps with other species.

So where in Hades did this devilishly clever DNA come from? The ultimate source may lie in the dirt beneath our feet.

For the past decade, Gerry Wright has been trying to understand the rise of drug resistance by combing through the world's richest natural source of resistance-enabling DNA: a clod of dirt. As the head of McMaster University's antibiotic research center in Hamilton, Ontario, Wright has the most tricked-out laboratory a drug designer could want, complete with a $15 million high-speed screening facility for simultaneously testing potential drugs against hundreds of bacterial targets. Yet he says his technology pales in comparison with the elegant antibiotic-making abilities he finds encoded in soil bacteria. The vast majority of the antibiotics stocking our pharmacy shelves—from old standards like tetracycline to antibiotics of last resort like vancomycin and, most recently, daptomycin—are derived from soil organisms.

Biologists assume that soil organisms make antibiotics to beat back the microbial competition and to establish their territory, Wright says, although the chemicals may also serve other, less-understood functions. Whatever the case, Wright and his students began combing through the DNA of soil microbes like streptomyces to better understand their impressive antibiotic-making powers. In doing so the researchers stumbled upon three resistance genes embedded in the DNA that *Streptomyces toyocaensis* uses to produce the antibiotic teicoplanin. While Wright was not surprised that the bug would carry such genes as antidotes to its own weaponry, he was startled to see that the antidote genes were nearly identical to the resistance genes in vancomycin-resistant enterococcus (VRE), the scourge of American and European hospitals.

"YET HERE THEY were in a soil organism, in the exact same orientation as you find in the genome of VRE," Wright says. "That sure gave us a head-slap moment. If only we had done this experiment 15 years ago, when vancomycin came into widespread use, we might have understood exactly what kind of resistance mechanisms would follow the drug into our clinics and hospitals." If nothing else, that foreknowledge might have prepared doctors for the inevitable resistance they would encounter soon after vancomycin was broadly prescribed.

Wright wondered what else he might find in a shovelful of dirt. So he handed out plastic bags to students departing on break, telling them to bring back soil samples. Over two years his lab amassed a collection that spanned the continent. It even included a thawed slice of tundra mailed by Wright's brother, a provincial policeman stationed on the northern Ontario-Manitoba border.

By 2005 Wright's team had combed through the genes of nearly 500 streptomyces strains and species, many never before identified. Every one proved resistant to multiple antibiotics, not just their own signature chemicals. On average, each could neutralize seven or eight drugs, and many could shrug off 14 or 15. In all, the researchers found resistance to every one of the 21 antibiotics they tested, including Ketek and Zyvox, two synthetic new drugs.

"These genes clearly didn't jump directly from streptomyces into disease-causing bacteria," Wright says. He had noted subtle variations between the resistance genes he pulled out of soil organisms and their doppelgängers in disease-causing bacteria. As in a game of telephone, each time a gene gets passed from one microbe to another, slight differences develop that reflect the DNA dialect of its new host. The resistance genes bedeviling doctors had evidently passed through many intermediaries on their way from soil to critically ill patients.

Wright suspects that the antibiotic-drenched environment of commercial livestock operations is prime ground for such transfer. "You've got the genes encoding for resistance in the soil beneath these operations," he says, "and we know that the majority of the antibiotics animals consume get excreted intact." In other words, the antibiotics fuel the rise of resistant bacteria both in the animals' guts and in the dirt beneath their hooves, with ample opportunity for cross-contamination.

Nobody knows how long free-floating DNA might persist in the water.

A 2001 study by University of Illinois microbiologist Roderick Mackie documented this flow. When he looked for tetracycline resistance genes in groundwater downstream from pig farms, he also found the genes in local soil organisms like Microbacterium and Pseudomonas, which normally do not contain them. Since then, Mackie has found that soil bacteria around conventional pig farms, which use antibiotics, carry 100 to 1,000 times more resistance genes than do the same bacteria around organic farms.

"These animal operations are real hot spots," he says. "They're glowing red in the concentrations and intensity of these genes." More worrisome, perhaps, is that Mackie pulled more resistance genes from his deepest test wells, suggesting that the genes percolated down toward the drinking water supplies used by surrounding communities.

An even more direct conduit into the environment may be the common practice of irrigating fields with wastewater from livestock lagoons. About three years ago, David Graham, a University of Kansas environmental engineer, was puzzled in the fall by a dramatic spike in resistance genes in a pond on a Kansas feedlot he was studying. "We didn't know what was going on until I talked with a large-animal researcher," he recalls. At the end of the summer, feedlots receive newly weaned calves from outlying ranches. To prevent the young animals from importing infections, the feedlot operators were giving them five-day "shock doses" of antibiotics. "Their attitude had been, cows are big animals, they're pretty tough, so you give them 10 times what they need," Graham says.

The operators cut back on the drugs when Graham showed them that they were coating the next season's alfalfa crop with highly drug-resistant bacteria. "Essentially, they were feeding resistance genes back to their animals," Graham says. "Once they realized that, they started being much more conscious. They still used antibiotics, but more discriminately."

While livestock operations are an obvious source of antibi-otic resistance, humans also take a lot of antibiotics—and their waste is another contamination stream. Bacteria make up about one-third of the solid matter in human stool, and Scott Weber, of the State University of New York at Buffalo, studies what hap-pens to the antibiotic resistance genes our nation flushes down its toilets.

Conventional sewage treatment skims off solids for landfill disposal, then feeds the liquid waste to sewage-degrading bacte-ria. The end result is around 5 billion pounds of bacteria-rich slurry, or waste sludge, each year. Around 35 percent of this is incinerated or put in a landfill. Close to 65 percent is recycled as fertilizer, much of it ending up on croplands.

WEBER IS NOW investigating how fertilizer derived from human sewage may contribute to the spread of antibiotic-resistant genes. "We've done a good job designing our treatment plants to reduce conventional contaminants," he says. "Unfortunately, no one has been thinking of DNA as a contaminant." In fact, sewage treatment methods used at the country's 18,000-odd wastewater plants could actually affect the resistance genes that enter their systems.

Every tested strain in a dirt sample proved resistant to mul-tiple antibiotics.

Most treatment plants, Weber explains, gorge a relatively small number of sludge bacteria with all the liquid waste they can eat. The result, he found, is a spike in antibiotic-resistant organisms. "We don't know exactly why," he says, "but our find-ings have raised an even more important question." Is the jump in resistance genes coming from a population explosion in the resistant enteric, or intestinal, bacteria coming into the sewage plant? Or is it coming from sewage-digesting sludge bacteria that are taking up the genes from incoming bacteria? The answer is important because sludge bacteria are much more likely to thrive and spread their resistance genes once the sludge is discharged into rivers (in treated wastewater) and onto crop fields (as slurried fertilizer).

Weber predicts that follow-up studies will show the resistance genes have indeed made the jump to sludge bacteria. On a hopeful note, he has shown that an alternative method of sewage processing seems to decrease the prevalence of bacterial drug resistance. In this process, the sludge remains inside the treatment plant longer, allowing dramatically higher concentrations of bacteria to develop. For reasons that are not yet clear, this method slows the increase of drug-resistant bacteria. It also produces less sludge for disposal. Unfortunately, the process is expensive.

Drying sewage sludge into pellets—which kills the sludge bacteria—is another way to contain resistance genes, though it may still leave DNA intact. But few municipal sewage plants want the extra expense of drying the sludge, and so it is instead exported "live" in tanker trucks that spray the wet slurry onto crop fields, along roadsides, and into forests.

Trolling the waters and sediments of the Cache la Poudre, Storteboom and Pruden are collecting solid evidence to support suspicions that both livestock operations and human sewage are major players in the dramatic rise of resistance genes in our environment and our bodies. Specifically, they have found unnaturally high levels of antibiotic resistance genes in sediments where the river comes into contact with treated municipal wastewater effluent and farm irrigation runoff as it flows 126 miles from Rocky Mountain National Park through Fort Collins and across Colorado's eastern plain, home to some of the country's most densely packed livestock operations.

"Over the course of the river, we saw the concentration of resistance genes increase by several orders of magnitude," Pruden says, "far more than could ever be accounted for by chance alone." Pruden's team likewise found dangerous genes in the water headed from local treatment plants toward household taps.

Presumably, most of these genes reside inside live bacteria, but a microbe doesn't have to be alive to share its dangerous DNA. As microbiologists have pointed out, bacteria are known to scavenge genes from the spilled DNA of their dead.

"There's a lot of interest in whether there's naked DNA in there," Pruden says of the Poudre's waters. "Current treatment of drinking water is aimed at killing bacteria, not eliminating their DNA." Nobody even knows exactly how long such free-floating DNA might persist.

All this makes resistance genes a uniquely troubling sort of pollution. "At least when you pollute a site with something like atrazine," a pesticide, "you can be assured that it will eventually decay," says Graham, the Kansas environmental engineer, who began his research career tracking chemical pollutants like toxic herbicides. "When you contaminate a site with resistance genes, those genes can be transferred into environmental organisms and actually increase the concentration of contamination."

Taken together, these findings drive home the urgency of efforts to reduce flagrant antibiotic overuse that fuels the spread of resistance, whether on the farm, in the home, or in the hospital.

For years the livestock pharmaceutical industry has played down its role in the rise of antibiotic resistance. "We approached this problem many years ago and have seen all kinds of studies, and there isn't anything definitive to say that antibiotics in livestock cause harm to people," says Richard Carnevale, vice president of regulatory and scientific affairs at the Animal Health Institute, which represents the manufacturers of animal drugs, including those for livestock. "Antimicrobial resistance has all kinds of sources, people to animals as well as animals to people."

The institute's own data testify to the magnitude of antibiotic use in livestock operations, however. Its members sell an estimated 20 million to 25 million pounds of antibiotics for use in animals each year, much of it to promote growth. (For little-understood reasons, antibiotics speed the growth of young animals, making it cheaper to bring them to slaughter.) The Union of Concerned Scientists and other groups have long urged the United States to follow the European Union, which in 2006 completed its ban on the use of antibiotics for promoting livestock growth. Such a ban remains far more contentious in North America, where the profitability of factory-farm operations depends on getting animals to market in the shortest possible time.

ON THE OTHER hand, the success of the E.U.'s ban is less than clear-cut. "The studies show that the E.U.'s curtailing of these compounds in feed has resulted in more sick animals needing higher therapeutic doses," Carnevale says.

"There are cases of that," admits Scott McEwen, a University of Guelph veterinary epidemiologist who advises the Canadian government on the public-health implications of livestock antibiotics. At certain stressful times in a young animal's life, as when it is weaned from its mother, it becomes particularly susceptible to disease. "The lesson," he says, "may be that we would do well by being more selective than a complete ban."

McEwen and many of his colleagues see no harm in using growth-promoting livestock antibiotics known as ionophores. "They have no known use in people, and we see no evidence that they select for resistance to important medical antibiotics," he says. "So why not use them? But if anyone tries to say that we should use such critically important drugs as cephalosporins or fluoroquinolones as growth promoters, that's a no-brainer. Resistance develops quickly, and we've seen the deleterious effects in human health."

A thornier issue is the use of antibiotics to treat sick livestock and prevent the spread of infections through crowded herds and flocks. "Few people would say we should deny antibiotics to sick animals," McEwen says, "and often the only practical way to administer an antibiotic is to give it to the whole group." Some critics have called for restricting certain classes of critically important antibiotics from livestock use, even for treating sick animals. For instance, the FDA is considering approval of cefquinome for respiratory infections in cattle. Cefquinome belongs to a powerful class of antibiotic known as fourth-generation cephalosporins, introduced in the 1990s to combat hospital infections that had grown resistant to older drugs. In the fall of 2006, the FDA's veterinary advisory committee voted against approving cefquinome, citing concerns that resistance to this vital class of drug could spread from bacteria in beef to hospital superbugs that respond to little else. But the agency's recently adopted guidelines make it difficult to deny approval to a new veterinary drug unless it clearly threatens the treatment of a specific foodborne infection in humans. As of press time, the FDA had yet to reach a decision.

Consumers may contribute to the problem of DNA pollution whenever they use antibacterial soaps and cleaning products. These products contain the antibiotic-like chemicals triclosan and triclocarban and send some 2 million to 20 million pounds of the compounds into the sewage stream each year. Triclosan and triclocarban have been shown in the lab to promote resistance to medically important antibiotics. Worse, the compounds do not break down as readily as do traditional antibiotics. Rolf Halden, cofounder of the Center for Water and Health at Johns Hopkins University, has shown that triclosan and triclocarban show up in many waterways that receive treated wastewater— more than half of the nation's rivers and streams. He has found even greater levels of these two chemicals in sewage sludge destined for reuse as crop fertilizer. According to his figures, a typical sewage treatment plant sends more than a ton of triclocarban and a slightly lesser amount of triclosan back into the environment each year.

For consumer antibacterial soaps the solution is simple, Halden says: "Eliminate them. There's no reason to have these chemicals in consumer products." Studies show that household products containing such antibacterials don't prevent the spread of sickness any better than ordinary soap and water. "If there's no benefit, then all we're left with is the risk," Halden says. He notes that many European retailers have already pulled these products from their shelves. "I think it's only a matter of time before they are removed from U.S. shelves as well."

Consumers may contribute to the problem of DNA pollution whenever they use soaps and cleaning products containing antibiotic-like compounds.

Finally, there is the complicated matter of the vast quantity of antibiotics that U.S. doctors prescribe each year: some 3 million pounds, according to the Union of Concerned Scientists. No doctor wants to ignore an opportunity to save a patient from infectious disease, yet much of what is prescribed is probably unnecessary—and all of it feeds the spread of resistance genes in hospitals and apparently throughout the environment.

"Patients come in asking for a particular antibiotic because it made them feel better in the past or they saw it promoted on TV," says Jim King, president of the American Academy of Family Physicians. The right thing to do is to educate the patient, he says, "but that takes time, and sometimes it's easier, though not appropriate, to write the prescription the patient wants."

Curtis Donskey, chief of infection control at Louis Stokes Cleveland VA Medical Center, adds that "a lot of antibiotic overuse comes from the mistaken idea that more is better. Infections are often treated longer than necessary, and multiple antibiotics are given when one would work as well." In truth, his studies show, the longer hospital patients remain on antibiotics, the more likely they are to pick up a multidrug-resistant superbug. The problem appears to lie in the drugs' disruption of a person's protective microflora—the resident bacteria that normally help keep invader microbes at bay. "I think the message is slowly getting through," Donskey says. "I'm seeing the change in attitude."

Meanwhile, Pruden's students at Colorado State keep amassing evidence that will make it difficult for any player—medical, consumer, or agricultural—to shirk accountability for DNA pollution.

Late in the afternoon, Storteboom drives past dairy farms and feedlots, meatpacking plants, and fallow fields, 50 miles downstream from her first DNA sampling site of the day. Leaving her Jeep at the side of the road, she strides past cow patties and fast-food wrappers and scrambles down an eroded embankment of the Cache la Poudre River. She cringes at the sight of two small animal carcasses on the opposite bank, then wades in, steering clear of an eddy of gray scum. "Just gross," she mutters, grateful for her watertight hip boots.

Of course, the invisible genetic pollution is of greater concern. It lends an ironic twist to the river's name. According to local legend, the appellation comes from the hidden stashes (cache) of gunpowder (poudre) that French fur trappers once buried along the banks. Nearly two centuries later, the river's hidden DNA may pose the real threat.

Real Men Get Prostate Cancer

Dana Jennings

From the *New York Times*, "Well" blog

Hormone therapy to shrink or slow the growth of prostate cancer is one of the most common treatments for the disease. *New York Times* editor Dana Jennings, who was diagnosed with prostate cancer earlier this year, talks about his own treatment with the drug Lupron.

THE DAY AFTER my most recent hormone injection for prostate cancer, I told my wife, Deb, that I had a headache, hot flashes, cramps and was very, very hungry.

She said, "Sweetie, you're having your period." We both laughed. (Laughter is a crucial therapy in my treatment.)

Those are just a few of the side effects I've been experiencing on Lupron, which is part of the hormonal treatment for my advanced case of prostate cancer. Lupron is a testosterone suppressant, designed to starve hormone-dependent cancer cells of the fuel (testosterone) that they crave in order to grow. My doctors believe, and studies indicate, that using hormonal therapy to complement my radiation treatments, which are scheduled to start next month, will give me a better chance of being cured, of survival.

In the past couple weeks, I've also had back, joint and muscle aches, random itchiness: that spider-crawling-on-your-skin feeling, cotton mouth, sudden fatigue and fleeting bursts of pain in my jaw, chest and armpits. These are not complaints, just observations.

Oh, and my testicles are shrinking. There's also intermittent testicle tenderness and, sometimes, they get so warm they feel as if they're on simmer. And the most unexpected side effect, so far, is that sometimes during sex, a Lupron headache suddenly descends and hammers at my skull.

Essentially, my Lupron shots are inducing biochemical (but reversible) castration. Besides the hot flashes and shrinking testicles, another potential side effect is that a man's breasts grow larger and more sensitive. Now, I'll tell you straight up, no doctor ever sits you down and says, "Son, to cure you, we might have to kind of turn you into a woman." I suspect that some men would almost rather die than have hot flashes and larger breasts.

These facts home in on why so many men often have trouble talking about prostate cancer. The treatment of the disease strikes at the very heart of our clichéd, John Wayne image of the American male. Impotence and incontinence, cramps and man-breasts just don't sell pickup trucks and the King of Beers, hoss. These symptoms are not some mere midlife crisis—more like a change-of-life crisis—that can be salved or solved with topical (and typical) macho palliatives, like buying a candy-apple-red Hummer or having an extramarital affair. They shake the very pillars of what we talk about when we talk about being a man.

I'm trying to cope with my prostate cancer, its treatment and its retinue of emasculating side effects by gathering myself each morning, seeking the man I still am—that I know I am—in the steamy bathroom mirror, and swearing to love all the things I love in this sweet old world more than ever: My wife and my sons, my faith, and my friends (and classic soul and country music).

I refuse to become my side effects and have decided that side effects are only side effects, a dark but necessary door to walk through toward the possibility of being well. And, hey, at least my voice is still deep.

Other common side effects of Lupron include lessened sexual desire (not yet, in my case), impotence (it depends on your definition) and osteoporosis—I'm taking a calcium supplement twice a day and walking miles and miles to try to prevent that.

When it comes to my current side effects, the hot flashes are the strangest—and, literally, keep me awake at night. Sometimes, they feel like an unusually warm spring day creeping up my back. Other times, they're like being jammed into a stuffed New York City subway car in August, and the air-conditioning is broken. My healthy red glow? Chemically induced.

So, on any given Sunday this fall, you'll find me nesting on the couch with my 22-year-old son, Drew, crunching on salty snacks (I told you that I was very, very hungry), nursing the one porter or stout I treat myself to, and watching the N.F.L.—my face flushed with the occasional hot flash, and "kegeling" all the while. You women remember kegeling—the contracting and relaxing of the muscles that make up the pelvic floor, exercises recommended before and after pregnancy. Well, prostate cancer patients need to do them, too, mainly to help improve bladder control.

It's true. Real men—even when they're on Lupron—can kegel and watch the N.F.L. at the same time.

10 Lessons of Prostate Cancer

Prostate cancer is a dark waltz, not the raging battle of popular imagination. From that first elevated PSA blood test, to the biopsy, to treatment, to those evil twins of impotence and incontinence and beyond, I'm still learning some very complicated steps more than seven months after my diagnosis.

Cancer is a hard teacher. No matter how much you glean from the Web, how many fellow travelers you talk to, how many

questions you ask nurses and doctors, there are some lessons—
physical, practical, emotional—that can only be learned
firsthand.

I confess that I feel utterly vulnerable. But, as the poet Theo-
dore Roethke wrote, "Those who are willing to be vulnerable
move among the mysteries." So, as I continue to move among
these mysteries, here are 10 nuggets of prostate cancer wisdom
that I had to learn for myself.

1. Cancer takes you home. The hardest thing I've
   had to do since my diagnosis—and that includes
   having my radical open prostatectomy—was tell
   my parents that I had prostate cancer. My folks are
   working-class country people. They're both 68, and
   they were 17 when I was born in 1957—eight days
   after they got married. The three of us, literally,
   grew up together, and I've always been their little
   hyper-verbal mystery. They never quite understood
   why I needed to get the hell out of Kingston, N.H.
   And when I called them last April to say that I had
   cancer—maybe, after all these years, confirming
   their worst fears about life in and around New
   York City—I could barely speak for my fierce tears.
   Tears more for them, I know, than for me.

2. Doctors forget to share the gory details. After my
   prostate was removed, my testicles swelled to the
   size of shot-puts—bright, red shot-puts—and stayed
   that way for days. Nobody told me to expect this
   condition, and only ice brought relief. (Conversely,
   now that I'm undergoing hormonal therapy, my
   testicles are shrinking.)

3. Insurance can cause more stress than cancer. The
   goal of your insurer—no matter how singular or
   complex your case is—is to try to turn you into a
   statistical cliché, a cipher, in the face of your very

human flesh-and-blood disease. In the months after my diagnosis, as my wife and I struggled to find the right pair of highly-skilled hands to perform my potentially difficult surgery, wrestling with my insurer caused me more grief, stress and depression than my cancer did. In our modern health-care-industrial-complex—and I'm talking about the bureaucrats who try to herd you into the cheapest cattle car available, not the nurses and doctors who are on the front lines—the emphasis is neither on health nor care, but on the bottom line. It's our job, as patients, to resist with all our strength.

4. Humor is all around you. On Halloween morning my wife and I were driving to the Cancer Institute of New Jersey in New Brunswick for my treatment. Just a quarter-mile from the institute we were stuck in traffic behind a truck . . . a casket truck: "Batesville Casket Company," it read, "A Hillen-brand industry, helping families honor the lives of those they love." All I could do was laugh harder than I had in days. (On a different drive down, the Beatles' "Do You Want to Know a Secret" came on the radio, and I dissolved into tears. I still don't understand why.)

5. Not all blood techs are created equal. Some glide that needle into your vein as if they're figure-skating on your arm. Others jab and stab as if they got their only training from watching the "Saw" movies. (By the way, only blood is "blood red.")

6. Nurses know what you need. I groaned in absolute gratitude in the recovery room at the post-op ice chips the nurses spooned into my swollen, anesthe-sia-parched mouth.

7. Cancer can be a punch line. I learned pretty
   quickly, with my wife and sons, that the phrase,
   "I've got cancer," wasn't a bad punch line—as in:
   "You take out the dog. I've got cancer" or "You
   answer the phone. I've got cancer" or "I 'call' the
   TV to watch 'Monday Night Football.' I've got
   cancer." They'd all roll their eyes, laugh . . . then go
   do what I asked.

8. Home remedies are essential to cancer recovery.
   There is no better post-op therapy on a sweltering
   July day than a cold glass of lemonade, a tran-
   scendent oldie on the CD player—say, "Doggin'
   Around" by Jackie Wilson—a stack of comic books
   at hand ("The Incredible Hulk," "The Mighty
   Thor") and the grace of a funny and compassion-
   ate visitor.

9. Don't sneeze after surgery. My first post-op
   sneeze felt as if some beyond-feral wolverine had
   burrowed its way into my gut, possibly seeking
   a second prostate that the docs had somehow
   overlooked.

10. You can find hope in strange places. A few times
    a day, after my operation, I'd run my fingers up
    and down the 25 metal staples that the surgeon
    had used to close me up—the skin around them
    red-purple, proud, tender and feeling as if it
    belonged to someone else. Sometimes, in fingering
    those staples, I felt that they were the only things
    in this world, in their plain and utilitarian way, that
    were possibly holding me together.

I Want My Life Back

Andrea Coller

From Glamour

How does a sarcastic, tattooed, music-obsessed, Tic Tac-popping, vodka-drinking 27-year-old feel when her cancer comes back for the third time? Angry—and determined to come out alive. You'll be blown away by the winner of *Glamour's* fifth personal essay contest, gritty survivor Andrea Coller.

AM I DEAD? Did it happen? Did I die?

I can't move. I can't see. But I can hear. Clicking. Beeping. Footsteps. Unfamiliar voices. Cryptic loudspeaker announcements. Hospital noises. I try to listen to the voices, but they float in and out in waves. They talk a lot about urine flow. Sometimes they say my name.

No. I must still be in here, somewhere.

I'm thinking I'm in a coma. And I'm thinking it could be worse. A coma has its obvious drawbacks, but at least you get to catch up on your sleep. And if nothing else, it's a spectacular excuse for eavesdropping. The downside is, most of the conversations are about urine.

I sleep.

I wake up.

I hear the quick click of high heels from down the hall. Mom. They get closer and closer. I feel her presence beside me.

"Can she hear me?" Mom asks.

"Yup," the nurse says.

"I'm here, baby," she whispers.

I fall asleep, then wake to Dad's voice.

"Hey, Pat," he says to my mother.

"Hey," she says back. I hear him walk from the doorway to my bed.

"I didn't know she had a tattoo."

Jesus Christ, Dad, I try to say, but I can't. I'm not naked, am I?

"Oh, just the one, though," my mom says. "Very small and tasteful." Suddenly I think that if I ever wake up for good, I'm gonna get me a badass face tattoo. An awful one, maybe Yosemite Sam waving a NASCAR flag. I feel my Dad come closer.

I fall asleep again. I wake up to sad TV applause as an announcer pronounces the season over for the Red Sox.

Ugh. I need a drink.

"Yankees," another voice says, disgusted.

Hi, big brother. I try. Still no words.

Shit, this better not be permanent.

"Andrea," Mom whispers to me, "squeeze my hand."

OK, I tell my brain, do it. I command my brain to make my hand move. It doesn't happen. I try again. It doesn't happen. Frustration starts to simmer inside me.

I am not helpless. I do not do helpless.

I hear my mom and the nurse talking. They're bringing me out of the coma, but it's going to be gradual. I'm fighting the sleep, hard, but it wins again.

When I wake up, I can move my tongue. I start to feel that there's a big giant tube down my throat. I try to focus on moving something. Anything. Soon, I have my right index finger going.

I hear my mom and sister-in-law going over The Pampered Chef catalog.

Hey! I have another finger. Eventually my family starts to notice. I grit myself, like you'd grit your teeth, so hard you think you'll break them, and it all starts to come together.

My eyelids are lifting. I will the half-circles of white light in front of me to expand. Twin suns rise in front of me and slowly dissolve into each other.

I can see. My family is gathered around my bed. They look awful. I meet their eyes with urgency. I respond to the nurse's questions with shaky finger taps.

I am declared present enough to take the breathing tube out. It's a fight with the nurse, who keeps telling me to calm down. I don't want to calm down! She tells me she's not taking the tube out until I get my heart rate down. I try to concentrate.

Somehow, I calm myself. I vomit out the tube. I breathe heavy on my own.

They tell me not to try to talk. I try to talk, and it comes out like a blur, a wild, stringy blur. My family laughs.

Laugh all you want, folks. See if I change your diapers in 50 years.

Annoyed and exhausted, I sink back into the bed. The nurse holds up a board with letters and "important" phrases on it for me to point to. I look for "Diet Coke," "You all suck," "Starbucks" or "vodka" but don't find any of them. I see a question mark and aim for it but just end up knocking the board out of her hands.

I look at my mother and mouth, "What happened?"

"Well, you were at work, and you were coughing up blood again . . . ," she begins.

I know very well what happened there. I'm trying to forget.

"I know," I mouth.

She skips to the juicy part: A big blood vessel burst in my lung, and they put me in a coma in order to go in and cauterize it. "OK," I mouth slowly.

She puts her hand on mine, I can feel its warmth. I look down at my arm, which is weak and limp and still doesn't seem like my own.

"Do you know why you have a penny taped to your hospital bracelet?" she asks.

I think I can move my head. I try. Slow. Up. Down.

"Yes."

I remember.

A few days earlier. It's a slow day at the salon, and I'm taking a bathroom break.

Blood. No.

Suddenly, I find myself sitting on the toilet, leaning forward, coughing bright red blood into a wad of toilet paper.

No. No. I stand up, shakily, throw the toilet paper in the toilet, flush and exit the stall. I look in the mirror. My face is pale.

This is not me. This is not happening to me.

I try to take a deep breath but just cough into my hands. I look down, and they're spattered with blood. The sink is spattered as well. I wash my hands, my mouth, my nose. I clean the sink. I take a spare roll of toilet paper back into the salon with me and pick up the phone from its cradle.

One more time, and I'm calling Dr. Bowers, I tell myself. It happens. Twice, in rapid succession.

Shit.

I shakily dial Dr. Bowers' office. The receptionist answers.

"It's Andrea Coller. It's happening again. The bleeding," I say.

"OK, I'm getting Dr. Bowers."

Breathe. Try to breathe. I bring up blood again. A little more this time. I grab one of the grocery bags we throw trash in and use it for my growing collection of TP wads.

"Andrea?" she says. "Dr. Bowers says to go right to the emergency room and he'll meet you there."

I hang up. Call an ambulance? No. I think of the mortifica-
tion of having the paramedics drag me out of work in front of
my coworkers and the women getting their hair done. No. I dial
the phone again.

Please answer. Please answer.

"Hello?"

"Meredith? It's happening again. The blood. Can you take
me to the hospital? I'm at work. I'll wait outside."

"I'll be right there."

I grab my purse and walk out to the sidewalk. I'm leaning
against the building, holding my roll of toilet paper and trash
bag of bloody tissues, coughing fresh blood into my fist. Strangers walk by and give me long stares. After a few minutes, I see
Meredith's red Jetta speed up and pull over to a screeching halt.
I get in.

"Hi," I say.

"Hi, darlin'. It's gonna be OK," she says.

"I'm sorry," I say. I really am.

"For what?"

"Scaring you. Calling you in the middle of the day. Coughing up blood in your car." As I do it. Again.

"Well, I knew I was unemployed for a reason. And don't you
apologize to me."

"This sucks," I say. We keep hitting red lights. Kids are cross-
ing the street in front of us.

"It's gonna be OK," she says again. "Goddamn it, I promise
you I'd be mowing shit over if I could."

"I know."

We get to the E.R. a few minutes later. Meredith drops me
off while she parks the car. I walk in and go up to the window.
The triage nurse asks a few questions and starts to take my blood
pressure. I cough again. I open the tissue and show her.

"Bright red," she says, taking a breath. "OK, come on back here." She leads me to a room in the back.

Doctors come in. I use the words. I tell them that I have Hodgkin's disease, that I've been in remission twice, but now it's back. I tell them I've been to the E.R. once before for the same thing, coughing up blood, but that time it was less and had stopped before the paramedics had even gotten to me. I tell them that Dr. Bowers had surmised that the blood was the result of the tumor breaking away from the wall of my lung as the chemo had shrunk it. They listen—for once—then hook me up to an IV. They tell me I need to cough directly into a Baggie so that they can measure it. I start doing it. It looks like a lot.

Meredith comes in and finds me. I give her my cell phone and tell her to call my mother. She goes outside again.

Dr. Bowers arrives. It's been an hour or so, with no sign of letting up. The last episode lasted only 15 minutes.

"We've got to transfer you to Baystate," he says. "We can't stop the bleeding here."

"Oh," I say. The reality is starting to sink in: The bleeding won't stop on its own. They have to go in and stop it.

"I'm trying to reach your mom," he says. "I left a couple of messages."

"My friend is trying too," I say, gathering courage. "Dr. Bowers?"

"Yeah?"

"You always tell me the truth," I say.

"Yes."

Am I dying? I need to know.

"Is this it?" I ask. He looks down for a minute, then looks back at me.

"I don't know," he says. "But we're going to do our best."

"OK," I say. I'm not sure it's OK, but the absence of bullshit is strangely comforting.

"I'm going to go back and get on the phone with the doctors over at Baystate. And I'm going to make sure that they tell you the truth," he says.

"Thanks," I say.

Shit.

Meredith comes back. She sits down beside me.

"Hey, darlin'," she says. "So your mom is in Seattle on business, but she's going to get here as soon as she can."

"And," she adds, looking away from me, "I called Mark."

"What?"

"I had to."

"What?" I repeat. Wow, what do you do when you're coughing up blood and your best friend has just called your ex-boyfriend without your permission?

"What?" I say again.

She shrugs.

The nurse brings in a hospital gown. I realize that I'm sprawled out on the cot in my work clothes–chandelier earrings, full skirt and heels. Holding a bag of blood. Nice. I take off my clothes in between coughing fits. Meredith picks things up as I take them off and folds them neatly. Her red hair falls in front of her face, like it does when she leans over her guitar. I put the gown on, still wearing my bra and underwear. The nurse says I have to take those off too.

"How come?" I ask. I can't imagine what they're going to do to me that can't get done with my bits and pieces nicely covered.

The nurse shrugs and avoids answering. I manage to pull the Flashdance bra trick around my hospital gown. I shimmy out of my underwear. Meredith takes them and folds them, too.

Dr. Bowers comes back in. He tells me they have to put a catheter and a breathing tube in and they're going to knock me out. He holds out a penny to me.

"This is my lucky penny," he says, "and I'm giving it to you."

"OK," I say. This is a bad sign.

"But I want it back," he says. He looks at me over his glasses.

"Thanks," I say.

They bring in someone to knock me out. The needle goes into my spine. And it burns. I catch a glimpse of the breathing tube that they're going to put in. It's huge. Meredith has seen it too and has one of the doctors cornered. Her red hair starts to swim around her face, like she's underwater.

"You need to be careful, because she's a singer," she says. Her mostly veiled Southern accent peeks out from behind her words.

"Well, we're not worried about that right now. We're trying to save her life," the doctor says.

"I realize that, but you need to be careful!" she says. The doctor replies, but I can't make it out. The room goes wavy, like Meredith's hair, like ocean water.

I love you.

My eyes fall closed.

A nervous-looking intern wakes me up in the morning. He doesn't wear glasses, but looks like he used to. I'm thirsty as hell, and my throat is sore. I'm cranky. Hell, I just got out of a coma. He explains that they're going to call paramedics to take me to the radiation building to give a big blast of the stuff to my lung.

"And then I'm getting the hell out of here," I say, voice scratchy.

"Um," he says, looking over his shoulder at the nurse, "I don't know about that."

"So, good," I say, "it's settled. I'm getting the hell out of here." "I didn't say. . . ," he stammers, trying to get the nurse's attention. She does her best to stifle a smile.

"Look, get this tube," I say, pointing at my crotch, "out from all up in my lady business, OK?" My throat hurts from talking, but it's totally worth it. He mumbles something, then backs out of the room.

"He's totally pissing his pants right now," I whisper to the nurse.

She smiles at me, gives a near-imperceptible wink and leaves.

The paramedics arrive with a stretcher, ready to take me to radiation. And they're hot. Like soap opera paramedics. I must look like hell. This would happen to me.

"Hey, guys," I whisper hoarsely. "What's up?"

"We're driving you around the corner, to radiation," the tall one says.

"Sounds like a pretty boring call," I squeak. "Sorry about that."

"Hey, boring's good," the other one says. "Especially on a Friday."

Friday? Really? What's the last day I remember?

"Friday, huh?" I ask. "You boys going out tonight?"

They smile and look down as my mom walks in. They move toward the door.

"Mom, get out," I whisper. "I was trying to score."

"The short one's got a ring," she says. "And the tall one looks like trouble."

"So? God, Mom, why you gotta mess up my groove?"

"I just love you, is all," she says, and puts her hand on my forehead.

"Yeah," I say. "You're kind of the greatest."

The paramedics do their job, wave a polite goodbye and leave. At the radiation center, they matter-of-factly tattoo and irradiate me. The radiation oncologist tells me that I'll have to come back nearly every day for months.

I need to get out of here.

"So, Doctor, can you please report to the other doctors that I'm ready to get the hell out of here? Like now?"

"Well, that's not my decision," he says.

That's all you doctors do, is pass the fucking buck. I space out completely as he goes into the details of my treatment.

So what? It's always the same. I'm always going to die.

I get taken back to the ICU by decidedly less hot paramedics. The doctors tell me that, since I have improved, they're moving me. They're just waiting for a bed for me on the cancer floor.

"See, I just don't think you all have heard me," I shout. "I want out of here now!" My throat burns from raising my voice. I can't stay here. I need to wake up in my apartment. I need to get to work early and drink coffee at the reception desk before anyone else gets there. I need my friends. I need my life.

I will not cry for these assholes. I will not give them the satisfaction.

I don't cry. I never cry in front of doctors.

They grudgingly let me go home after another night spent stable in the hospital. My parents kick into crisis mode and stay with me for a few days. Mom fixes me macaroni and cheese with little hot dog pieces in it. Dad and I watch the Three Stooges. They both call me their "little girl."

I finish my radiation. I finish my chemo. Winter comes. I get shingles. I'm in and out of the hospital again. I fight. I can't breathe very well. I'm tired.

Spring comes, and I'm done. I get a clear CAT scan. For the third time in my life, I'm officially in remission. I go back to work full-time. I still can't breathe very well. I'm so tired.

Dr. Bowers and I try steroids, inhalers, inhaled steroids, antibiotics, and nothing really helps me to breathe better. Then he drops a bomb. The doctors at Dana-Farber whom he consults with have suggested another stem cell transplant. I'd had one already, during my second bout with cancer. It was unspeakably vile and did not work.

"Wait a minute," I say, confused. "I thought I was in remission here."

"It was expected to be temporary . . . ," he pauses. "What did they tell you?"

"My God, they are such assholes!"

"Well, they may be, but they know what they're doing," he says.

No. You're better than all of them put together. Times a million. Dr. Bowers hands me the small box of scratchy hospital tissues.

I must be crying. I can't be.

But I am.

"So . . . what happens if I just, like, ride this remission out?" I ask.

"The odds that you're cured from this course of treatment are not very good."

Radiation every day for weeks. Hours and hours spent in the chemo chair, watching poison drip into my veins. For nothing.

"How not good?" I ask. "Like virtually zero or more like 10 percent?"

"More like 10," he says.

"OK," I say, breathing in around the obstructions in my chest. "I'll take it."

I've had four CAT scans, one every three months for the last year. It's hard for the doctors to see much—with all of the scar tissue and screws and sponges and cigarette butts and banana peels left in there from the whole cauterization episode—but there have been no changes to the way the scan looks in about a year. If the next scan comes up clean, with no changes, it will be my longest remission yet.

The scarring in my lung takes the form of weeping wounds, which cause me to have a chronic cough. It's mostly manageable but sometimes comes in fits. When people ask about it, I usually blame it on allergies. Sometimes I like to mix it up and tell people I'm a recovering meth addict. On rare occasions I tell the truth. It slips out if I let my guard down, generally if I am disarmed by honest eyes or alcohol.

If I tell the truth, I'm called brave. People tell me that I must have so much perspective.

You don't want to hear my perspective.

They think that I must be all Zen. That I eat organic, drink wheatgrass and meditate. They think that I've gained an understanding about life, just from having spent so much time close to death.

Bullshit.

I'm decidedly non-Zen. I balance my diet with coffee and cocktails. And Tic Tacs. Don't forget the Tic Tacs. If anything, I am more messed up and confused about life than ever.

I am also too nice to shatter their illusions. Because when their mothers are diagnosed with breast cancer, when their kids get leukemia, they're going to want to think that at the end of all of the suffering, they will have the shining light of perspective. In truth, they will be lucky if they emerge with any memory of their former selves. That is the hardest part of all. I am trying to clear out a space in my mind around all of the shrapnel of the things I wish I could forget so that I can make way for the things I want to remember.

"Yes, I have a lot of perspective," I say.

"Pick-suhs."

It's my niece's second-birthday party, and I'm squatting with her in the driveway. She's caught me staring into space, my sidewalk chalk poised on the pavement.

"Pictures, right," I say. My voice is gravelly. This is my second birthday party in the past 24 hours. My friend Juliette's party the night before had been punctuated by my drunken vomiting at the bar, after I'd once again tried to drink the past five years under the table. She and her husband carried me out, drove me home and stayed with me while I puked several more times, showered, dry-heaved, cried and finally passed out on my bathroom floor at three in the morning.

That is not me. Please let them understand that is not me.

"Pick-suhs," my niece insists. Sorry, kid. Auntie's hung over.

I look up, and Rose has turned to get a different-color chalk.
In her tiny hand, it looks enormous. With an intense look of concentration, she draws a line, examines it and draws another.

I ruined Juliette's birthday.

"Pink!" Rose says.

"What's that?" I ask.

Just try.

"Spaghetti? Pink spaghetti?" I ask.

Just stop.

"Pink suh-get-tee!" she squeals and laughs. The sun glints
off her blond curls and her tiny white teeth.

"Pretty pick-suh," she says, nodding.

Stop.

I look down at the chalk, my hand holding it, her picture.
I follow Rose's gaze upward. I look at her. Her brown eyes find
me.

For a second.

I remember.

For just this second.

I remember who I am.

Going Under: A Doctor's Downfall, and a Profession's Struggle with Addiction.

Jason Zengerle

From the *New Republic*

IN DECEMBER 2003, Brent Cambron gave himself his first injection of morphine. Save for the fact that he was sticking the needle into his own skin, the motion was familiar–almost rote. Over the course of the previous 17 months, as an anesthesia resident at Boston's Beth Israel Deaconess Medical Center, Cambron had given hundreds of injections. He would stick a syringe into a glass ampule of fentanyl or morphine or Dilaudid, pulling up the plunger to draw his dose. Then he'd inject the dose into his patient. If the patient had been in a panic before her surgery, Cambron would watch her drift into a pleasant, happy daze; if the patient had been moaning in pain after surgery, he'd watch the relief spread across her face as the pain went away. It was understandable, perhaps, that Cambron was curious to experience these sensations himself, to feel what his patients felt once the drugs began coursing through their bodies. It could even be considered a clinical experiment of sorts. "I had thought about it for a long time," he later confessed.

The way in which Cambron handled his own injection reflected that intense curiosity—but also a degree of caution. Although Cambron had been a physician for less than two of his 30 years, in that brief time he'd acquired a fund of knowledge that left him certain he knew what he was doing. With his patients, he typically delivered drugs intravenously, so that the medicine went directly into their bloodstreams and its effects were immediate. Now that he was delivering the drug to himself, he injected it into his muscle; that way, the morphine would have to seep through layers of fat and tissue before it began to circulate through his system, resulting in a slower, less intense, and presumably safer high. An intravenous injection, as one of Cambron's fellow residents would say, is like "putting fuel on a fire," but an intramuscular injection "is like putting a cookie in your mouth and letting it soak, so that you're not really chewing it and it's not getting into your stomach."

Cambron initially told no one of his decision to use morphine—not his colleagues, not even his live-in girlfriend, from whom he hid his syringes. What he was doing was illegal, and he knew others would disapprove. But his shame was leavened by a certain amount of confidence, even arrogance. During the 80-hour weeks he put in at Beth Israel, a Harvard teaching hospital considered one of the best in the world, he practiced medicine at its highest level. People could quibble with other choices Cambron might make, but if he chose to do something medical—even to himself—then it was, by definition, the right choice.

That first injection of morphine, however, would quite possibly be the last time Cambron actually chose to do drugs. As the needle broke the skin and the morphine slowly seeped into his system that December day, Cambron began to cede control over his own medical powers. Before long, his career—and much more—would be in jeopardy.

THE COMMON CONCEPTION of anesthesiologists is that they do little more than put people to sleep while surgeons perform the true medical miracles. The reality of their job is more complicated—not to mention harrowing. In the course of putting a patient under, the anesthesiologist must maintain the patient's delicate physiological balance. Because the drugs he uses to put a patient to sleep often lower the person's heart rate and blood pressure, the anesthesiologist must administer other drugs to raise them. If the surgery requires silencing the patient's brain and paralyzing his muscles, then the anesthesiologist must control the patient's breathing, since the patient can no longer do so himself. During a surgery, in short, the anesthesiologist essentially takes over the patient's basic life-preservation functions.

As frightening as this process sounds, it routinely enables patients to undergo complex surgical procedures safely and without physical pain. Before the mid-nineteenth century, when anesthesia began to emerge as a medical specialty, this was rarely the case. Limbs were amputated and teeth extracted while patients were sentient and awake. Typical is a story recounted by a nineteenth-century Boston surgeon who helped treat a young man with tongue cancer: "The cancerous end . . . was cut off by a sudden, swift stroke of the knife, and then a red-hot iron was placed on the wound to cauterize it. Driven frantic by the pain and the sizzle of searing flesh inside his mouth, the young man escaped his restraints in an explosive effort and had to be pursued until the cauterization was complete, with his lower lip burned in the process."

Among the doctors troubled by the pain and suffering he caused his patients was a young Connecticut dentist named Horace Wells. In December 1844, Wells attended a performance by Gardner Quincy Colton, a one-time medical student who had become a sort of scientific showman. Colton invited a volunteer from the audience to place in his mouth a wooden faucet connected to a rubber bag of nitrous oxide. After inhaling the gas, Colton's volunteer ran around the theater like a wild man, gashing his leg in the process. What intrigued Wells, according to Henry W. Erving's *The Discoverer of Anesthesia: Dr. Horace Wells of Hartford*, was that the volunteer seemed impervious to pain. As it happened, Wells needed to have his wisdom tooth removed. The next day, he had Colton give him a dose of nitrous oxide, after which one of Wells's colleagues performed the extraction. "I didn't feel it so much as the prick of a pin!" Wells reported. He went on to give nitrous oxide to more than a dozen patients, storing the gas in an animal bladder and then asking them to suck it into their mouths via a wooden tube while he held their nostrils shut.

A few years later, after some setbacks with nitrous oxide, Wells began to experiment with chloroform as an anesthetic. As with nitrous oxide, he experimented on himself. This time, though, Wells developed an addiction to it—which sent him into a downward spiral. At the age of 33, after being arrested, he inhaled some chloroform and then with a razor severed his femoral artery, bleeding to death.

Today, anesthesiology has obviously come a long way from Wells's animal bladder of laughing gas. But, for all its technological advances, the specialty is still plagued by an addiction problem among its practitioners. In 1987, the addiction medicine doctor G. Douglas Talbott reviewed the files of 1,000 M.D.s who had enrolled in the Medical Association of Georgia's Impaired Physicians Program. He wanted to know how the drug-addicted physicians broke down by age, gender, and, most importantly, medical specialty. What Talbott discovered, and subsequently published in the *Journal of the American Medical Association*, was disturbing: Although anesthesiologists made up only 5 percent of the physician population, they accounted for 13 percent of those physicians being treated for drug addiction. The numbers Talbott found for younger physicians were even worse: While anesthesia residents constituted 4.6 percent of all resident physicians, they accounted for 33.7 percent of residents in treatment for drug addiction.

No studies have found a correlation between the addiction rate and medical error (although in 2002, a 31-year-old Washington State woman suffered severe brain damage after her anesthesiologist, who was addicted to Demerol, allegedly mismanaged her care during a routine surgical procedure). But Talbott's article served as a wake-up call to the specialty nonetheless. In the 20 years since its publication, anesthesia departments have worked to educate their members about the risk of addiction; they've become more vigilant about monitoring access and use of drugs by members; and some have even instituted mandatory urine tests for practitioners.

And yet, the problem has persisted. A 2005 study that surveyed more than 100 anesthesiology residency programs found that, between 1991 and 2001, 80 percent of them had physicians who became addicted to drugs during their training, and nearly 20 percent reported one death due to overdose or suicide. "We've gone through lots of steps to try to make it harder and harder, and that hasn't seemed to have had a lot of impact," says Keith Berge, an anesthesiologist at the Mayo Clinic in Minnesota who sits on the American Society of Anesthesiologists (ASA) Committee on Occupational Health. "Addiction," a recent article in the ASA's journal *Anesthesiology* concluded, "is still considered by many to be an occupational hazard for those involved in the practice of anesthesia."

WHEN BRENT CAMBRON arrived in Boston in the summer of 2002 to start his residency at Beth Israel Deaconess Medical Center, he could legitimately claim to be one of the top young anesthesia doctors in the country—and that was before he'd even handled his first case. Anesthesia is considered one of the most competitive specialties, and the program at Beth Israel, with its Harvard affiliation, was even more rarefied. It selected just twelve residents that year, and those it chose were invariably at or near the top of their med school classes.

That was certainly true of Cambron, a handsome young doctor with close-cut brown hair, gentle green eyes, and a thin, athletic build. But in other ways he didn't fit the typical Beth Israel anesthesia resident profile. Unlike many of his colleagues, who hailed from major metropolitan areas on the coasts, Cambron had grown up in the no-stoplight town of Sperry, Oklahoma, about 15 miles north of Tulsa, the son of a data processor and a homemaker. After scoring off the charts on his ACT test and graduating as his high school class's valedictorian, he attended the University of Oklahoma on a scholarship, matriculating to the University of Oklahoma College of Medicine. From his days in Sperry to his time in med school, Cambron had always sailed to the head of the class with ease. "There were some people who had to put in fourteen hours or so to learn the material, but it always seemed like Brent could do it in about seven," recalls Matthew Paden, a medical school classmate. "People would be incredibly stressed out and sleep-deprived and pepped up on coffee, and then he'd come walking down the hall with a smile on his face on his way to ride his bike."

And yet, despite his whiz-kid status, Cambron seemed happiest when he came off as ordinary. "You kind of had to know him for a while to know how smart he was," says his college roommate John E. Thomas. "He didn't flaunt it." Although he was a gifted musician, the outlet he chose for his musical talents was a college party cover band called Hummer. Even in that, he was content to stay in the background, playing rhythm guitar and singing backup. "Brent was very much a behind-the-scenes, below-the-radar kind of guy," says James Suliburk, one of Cambron's bandmates who also went to college and med school with him.

When it came time to do his residency, Cambron chose anesthesia, which would provide him with good pay, reasonable hours, and plenty of intellectual and emotional challenges.

In their need for constant vigilance, anesthesiologists are frequently likened to airline pilots: Both jobs entail long periods of boredom punctuated by moments of extreme terror. "From the moment you walk in the hospital until the moment you leave, you're waiting for disaster to happen, " says Ethan Bryson, an anesthesiologist at Mount Sinai hospital in New York. "And [when it does], you have to be ready to immediately intervene, recognize what's going on, and fix it, because someone's life depends on it."

As low-key as he liked to appear, Cambron craved this type of pressure. "If something was going to be difficult," says Thomas, "Brent always took it on." While most of his medical school classmates chose to do their residencies in Oklahoma, he decided to travel the great geographic and mental distance to Beth Israel.

Cambron immediately took to Boston. He rented an apartment on bustling Newbury Street, right in the heart of the ritzy Back Bay neighborhood, and attended concerts and Red Sox games. At the same time, he proved to be an excellent fit for Beth Israel. Even among the first-year residents, who typically work slavish hours, Cambron stood out for his penchant to get to the hospital early and leave late—something one fellow resident attributed to his "Midwestern work ethic." More importantly, during thelong hours he spent at the hospital, he impressed his colleagues with his clinical skills. "Sometimes a resident isn't born with what we call the 'oh shit gene' to recognize that something with a patient is quickly deteriorating," says Anthony Hapgood, a former Beth Israel anesthesia resident who was in the class ahead of Cambron's. "Brent wasn't like that. He could recognize when something was going wrong. He treated it early, and he treated it appropriately."

Cambron soon developed a reputation for levelheadedness during those moments of extreme terror—a levelheadedness that was rare not only in residents, but in more senior anesthesiologists, as well. Vivian Jung Tanaka, another of Cambron's co-residents, remembers the masterful way Cambron "ran codes"—medical jargon for leading the effort to resuscitate someone who's stopped breathing. "He was one of those unusual people that, no matter what happened, he kept his cool," she says. His placid demeanor was matched with a burning intelligence. "I think the first two years, he got the highest score on the practice board exam," says Suzanne Harrison, who was in Cambron's resident class.

In July 2004, Cambron's fellow residents and senior colleagues selected him to serve as a chief resident, one of the highest honors a junior physician can receive. By the time he received that honor, Cambron had been giving himself injections of morphine, fentanyl, and Dilaudid for nearly eight months.

THE DRUGS MOST frequently used in anesthesia today—such as the opioids fentanyl and Dilaudid, as well as the sedative propofol—are among the most potent in the history of medicine. Dilaudid and fentanyl, for instance, are eight and 100 times more potent than morphine, respectively. These drugs aren't only powerful, they're also extremely addictive. Because they are chemically engineered to have short half-lives, so that their effects do not linger and patients can be safely discharged sooner after their surgeries, recreational users of such drugs quickly develop heightened tolerances to them, meaning that they have to use more and more of the drugs in order to achieve their desired highs. "There's a crash-and-burn phenomenon with these drugs," says Paul Earley, the medical director of the Talbott Recovery Campus in Atlanta, which specializes in treating impaired physicians. "Whereas an alcoholic physician or one who's abusing oral narcotics might not manifest obvious signs of addiction for years or even decades, it's common for anesthesiologists to show up in treatment six months or nine months or a year after their first time taking one of these drugs."

Cambron was no stranger to recreational drug use. According to a journal he kept, he was a heavy drinker in college and in medical school; he also occasionally smoked marijuana. But maintaining a hard-partying lifestyle in the midst of an ambitious academic career seemed like the type of challenge that Cambron thrived on. "We would go out and party all night and do the things college kids do," recalls one of Cambron's college friends, "and then he'd get up the next day and study for an hour and go take a midterm and ace it." When Cambron arrived in Boston for his residency, he cut back on his alcohol consumption. Soon, though, Cambron began to go out drinking on weekends with some of the people in his program. In December 2002, he found a resident who did cocaine and the two began using together. When his co-resident couldn't get cocaine, they would snort powdered Ritalin. In the year before he began injecting himself with opioids, Cambron was drinking three or four nights a week and using cocaine once or twice a month. Ironically, once he tried the morphine, he liked it in part because it allowed him to drink less.

When Cambron was appointed chief resident, it seemed to strengthen his conviction that, when it came to his drug use, he knew what he was doing. "I felt that things must be going well since everyone thought I was doing well," he later wrote in his journal. Not long after becoming chief, when Cambron began having trouble with his girlfriend (who had moved with him to Boston from Oklahoma), he increased the doses, along with the frequency, of his opioid injections. And the frequency increased even further after Cambron and his girlfriend broke up about halfway through his one-year term as chief. He started spending more time socially with the residents he supervised—including one, he discovered, who also took intramuscular injections of morphine. They began doing the drugs together. In January 2006, the resident revealed to Cambron that she had started taking the drugs intravenously. Soon he was giving himself regular i.v. injections of morphine, fentanyl, and Dilaudid and occasional injections of propofol.

For a time, Cambron was able to manage his drug use as he had in the past. Indeed, in July 2006, after he completed a fellowship in pain medicine, Beth Israel hired him as an attending physician and he became a clinical instructor of anesthesiology at Harvard Medical School. But, before long, the i.v. injections left him with cravings that he could only satisfy with ever larger and ever more frequent doses. It became harder for him to conceal what he was doing, and his work began to suffer. On one occasion, he fell after giving himself an injection of propofol, splitting open his forehead and leaving him with a black eye. The doctor who once got to work early and left late was now getting to work late and leaving early. Some of his colleagues told him he looked "disheveled."

In December, a senior physician approached Cambron and asked if he would meet with her after grand rounds the next day. When Cambron looked at the schedule, he realized that the grand rounds speaker was the director of the Massachusetts Medical Society's Physician Health Services, a group that assists physicians struggling with drug addiction. Cambron knew what was coming, but he came up with a plan. His resident friend— who had recently returned from an unsuccessful three-month stay at the Betty Ford clinic—had obtained clean urine for her own regular drug tests. He took some of her supply to work with him the next day. And when, after grand rounds, he was confronted with suspicions that he was using drugs, he agreed to produce a urine sample.

But Cambron could only avoid getting caught for so long. He continued to use more and more frequently, injecting himself before work and then taking syringes to use at the hospital. By the end of January, he was giving himself i.v. injections of Dilaudid throughout his days at the hospital and slurring his words for the five or so minutes after each hit. Officials at Beth Israel wouldn't comment on exactly how or when they discovered Cambron was using drugs, citing hospital policy not to discuss personnel matters, but, in early February, Cambron took a leave from the hospital to enter a rehabilitation facility in Virginia that specializes in treating impaired physicians.

ON THE NIGHT of July 3, 2007, Cambron put on blue hospital scrubs, rented a Zipcar, and drove 20 miles from the Back Bay to a hospital in the suburban town of Norwood, where he'd once done some part-time work. Four weeks earlier, he'd returned to Boston from the Virginia rehab facility. He was sober and committed to recovery—and to going back to his old job at Beth Israel. Although this would seem akin to, as one anesthesiologist friend of Cambron's put it, "sending an alcoholic to work in a bar," it is actually not uncommon. Anesthesiology residents who become addicted and successfully complete recovery are often then redirected toward lower-risk medical specialties. But those anesthesiologists who have finished their training (as Cambron had) are more typically permitted to return to the specialty, so long as they are monitored by an impaired-physicians program— something Cambron had agreed to.

But, not long after getting back to Boston, Cambron was summoned to a meeting at Beth Israel with the hospital vice president and the chair of the anesthesia department, during which they asked him to resign from the hospital staff and agree to a voluntary suspension of his license. (Cambron's resident friend had earlier agreed to these same conditions, although her medical license was ultimately revoked.) Cambron acqui-esced, but he was devastated. "I felt betrayed by the people who were to have supported me," he wrote in his journal. A week or so later, Cambron snuck into Beth Israel, stole some propofol, and returned to his apartment, where he injected himself.

Now, as Cambron walked into the mostly empty Norwood hospital—his scrubs concealing the fact that he was, at that moment, prohibited from practicing medicine—he was once again determined to get sober. He carried with him used needles and some of his old supplies. He was going to throw them away. Even in the throes of addiction, he was still a physician and was a stickler when it came to the disposal of hazardous materials. "He was worried someone would get hurt going through the garbage," says Margaret Yoh, a Boston woman who was Cambron's girlfriend. But Cambron couldn't resist temptation. He swiped some propofol from an operating room, locked himself in a bathroom near the endoscopy unit, and injected the drug into his femoral artery. Before long a cleaning woman tried to gain entrance to the bathroom, but Cambron wouldn't come out. When he finally emerged over an hour later, hospital security officers were waiting for him. They noticed the blood on his hand, on his scrubs, and on the bathroom floor; they also noticed that Cambron was acting like, as one of them later put it, he was "on something." The security officers called the police. Cambron told them that he'd come to Norwood to pick up a bag for an anesthesiologist friend; the blood stains on his scrubs, he explained, were old. "I don't know why you keep questioning me," he protested. "This is no big deal." When they asked to search his backpack he refused. He was placed under arrest for trespassing and the officers then went through his bag, discovering a veritable pharmacy. He was charged with larceny and drug possession. At the police station, one of the officers asked Cambron if he was sick or injured. He told them he had the "disease of addiction." "To what?" the officer asked. "To everything," Cambron replied.

Cambron's father and his sister Kelly flew from Oklahoma to Boston to bail him out of jail. Kelly stayed at Cambron's apartment over the next several weeks to look after him. With a c.v. that now included a failed stint in rehab and an arrest record, Cambron seemed to have lost everything. But his medical license was still only suspended, not revoked, and he continued to hold out hope he could eventually return to anesthesia. He begged his sister to help him understand why he felt the need to use drugs in the first place. "He'd ask me if something went wrong in his childhood that he felt he'd need them," Kelly recalls. "I tried to help him figure that out and I couldn't. He was looking for any kind of reason for why he'd feel he needed them, because he couldn't figure it out, and it really bothered him."

THE ANESTHESIA SPECIALTY has been struggling with this question itself: Why do so many of its members suffer from addiction? The simplest—and most popular—explanation is access. Anesthesia is the only medical specialty in which physicians draw up, label, and account for their own drugs. As such, they have more opportunities than other physicians to abuse those drugs. "Anesthesiologists are left alone with open ampules of highly potent narcotics," explains Berge, "and it's easy to divert for their own use." Cambron was proof of that. Beth Israel Deaconess Medical Center, according to its vice president for education Richard Schwartzstein, has multiple policies and procedures in place to prevent such diversion—including the requirement that anesthesiologists "waste" whatever drugs they don't use on a patient in front of a witness or that they return the unused drugs to the pharmacy, which are then verified through random tests. But these safeguards proved no match for a determined addict like Cambron. "Addicts are smart, we're smart; they're desperate, we're not desperate," says Berge. "So they're going to outsmart us every time."

In recent years, however, the access hypothesis has started to be questioned. Its leading critic is Mark Gold, a psychiatrist and the former chief of addiction medicine at the University of Florida's McKnight Brain Institute. "If it's just holding the drugs," says Gold, "the pharmacists have the drugs, so do drug-abuse researchers, and not many of them become drug abusers or drug dependent." In 2004, Gold presented an alternative hypothesis to explain anesthesiology's addiction problem: exposure. Using gas chromatography-mass spectroscopy equipment, Gold had researchers scour several working operating rooms for traces of anesthetic agents. Sure enough, even though the anesthetics were administered intravenously, the researchers found throughout the operating rooms trace amounts of fentanyl and propofol, which the patients had exhaled. The highest concentrations were found around the patients' heads—which is where the anesthesiologists typically sit during surgeries. Gold, who did some of the pioneering work on secondhand cigarette addiction during the 1990s, had his new hypothesis. "It wasn't a great leap," he explains, "to say, possibly, that some number of anesthesiologists who become drug abusers and drug-addicted may have as an important contributory factor exposure to secondhand drugs in the O.R. Their brains changed in response to the secondhand drugs, and they developed cravings as if they were taking the drugs themselves."

Most anesthesiologists and other addiction experts doubt exposure can explain the problem, since the amounts of anesthetics found in the operating room are so miniscule. "I think it's invoking an incredibly complex explanation for something that has a much more simple explanation," says Berge. And yet, even many of those who subscribe to the access hypothesis concede that it's unsatisfying. "I agree that access has something to do with it," says one anesthesiologist, "but people have to want to take advantage of that access. There has to be some other explanation."

CAMBRON'S ARREST STARTED him on a vicious cycle of recovery and relapse. Over the next year, he would make numerous, serial attempts to get sober—again at the treatment facility in Virginia, at McLean Hospital outside Boston, and at a retreat in rural Connecticut that was started by Alcoholics Anonymous co-founder Bill Wilson. In each instance (including after he was arrested a second time, at Beth Israel), he would become sober for a while, before eventually, inevitably relapsing. In this, he was hardly unique. One 1990 study found that two-thirds of opioid-addicted anesthesiology residents who returned to their programs relapsed. Their continued access to drugs was surely a contributing factor, but there was something else that seemed to prevent their recovery.

The first of the twelve steps to sobriety is for the addict to admit that he is powerless over his addiction. The second step is to believe that a power greater than himself could restore him to sanity. But admitting this sort of powerlessness flies in the face of what makes someone a good anesthesiologist to begin with. Some anesthesiologists and addiction medicine specialists like to talk about what they call the "AOA disease"—referring to the Alpha Omega Alpha medical society, a sort of Phi Beta Kappa for med school students. Because only the top medical students are able to enter anesthesia residencies, it's a specialty stocked with overachievers. "They're driven and they don't know how to take care of themselves well, they're too compulsive about their work, they can't let cases go, they're almost wound too tight," Earley says of anesthesiologists. "And then, when the drug comes along, they just feel like, ahhhhhhhhh, I can finally relax. And it's in that experience that the setup for continued use occurs. If you've been wound tight all your life, the first time you use narcotics, you say to yourself, this is how normal people must feel." Raymond Roy, the chair of the anesthesiology department at Wake Forest University School of Medicine, relates some black humor that has made the rounds in anesthesia circles: "How can you avoid having any substance abusers in your residency? Recruit from the bottom of your med school class."

Compounding the problem is the fact that anesthesiology doesn't only draw overachievers but overachievers who, in order to succeed in the specialty, must also be control freaks—and, in particular, control freaks about drugs and the human body. "So much of what we do as a physician and as a specialist is control someone else's physiology," says Bryson. "We give what would be equivalent to a lethal injection on a daily basis if we didn't intervene. A lot of what we do is controlling the body's reaction to drugs. And I think that creates a false sense that, if we can control what's going on with somebody else, we should be able to control this in ourselves."

Cambron certainly seemed to suffer from that delusion. "He always told me that when he was taking these drugs, he knew exactly what he was doing," says his sister Kelly, "that whenever he messed around with stuff, because of his medical knowledge, he knew how much to do without going overboard."

SOMETIME IN THE night on October 13 or in the early morning hours of October 14, 2008, Cambron returned to the surgical suite on the third floor of the Beth Israel Deaconess Medical Center's Shapiro building. Once, the nine operating rooms there had been his professional home, where he'd work on knee repairs and breast biopsies and cataract surgeries. Now, they were simply a place where he could get drugs. Because the surgical suite in the Shapiro building was reserved for outpatient procedures, Cambron knew it would be empty at night. As he walked through the maze of hallways and through a series of imposing double doors, no one challenged his presence.

Cambron assembled his stash: It included five syringes, a 50-milligram vial of Demerol, four ten-milligram bottles of morphine, four ten-milligram bottles of Dilaudid, and a ten-milligram bottle of vecuronium—a muscle relaxant that, taken at high doses, will cause respiratory arrest in a matter of minutes. He brought all of it into a small room that bore the label "soiled utility" and was used to clean anesthesia equipment, closed the door, and began to inject himself.

At about 7:30 A.M., an anesthesia technician, who was making her morning rounds before the day's first surgery, opened the door. Cambron was sprawled on the floor between two stainless steel wash basins, his body surrounded by needles and empty vials, including, most ominously, the ten-milligram bottle of vecuronium. The technician ran for help and a team of doctors crowded into the small room. There was nothing they could do. At 7:47 A.M., a Beth Israel Deaconess anesthesiologist pronounced his former colleague dead. Cambron was 35 years old.

Two months later, with his death still under investigation by the police department, Cambron's friends and family don't know whether he meant to kill himself or whether his overdose was accidental. He left no suicide note, and he gave no signs that he was contemplating such an act. Indeed, he had recently arranged his apartment so that his girlfriend Yoh could move some of her things in. But the empty bottle of vecuronium is a haunting goodbye. After all, in spite of everything else that had gone wrong in his life, Cambron was an excellent doctor. Some of those who knew him have a hard time believing that he could have made such an elementary—and catastrophic—medical mistake.

Superbugs: The New Generation of Resistant Infections Is Almost Impossible to Treat

Jerome Groopman

From the *New Yorker*

Doctors fear that dangerous bacteria may become entrenched in hospitals.

IN AUGUST, 2000, Dr. Roger Wetherbee, an infectious-disease expert at New York University's Tisch Hospital, received a disturbing call from the hospital's microbiology laboratory. At the time, Wetherbee was in charge of handling outbreaks of dangerous microbes in the hospital, and the laboratory had isolated a bacterium called *Klebsiella pneumoniae* from a patient in an intensive-care unit. "It was literally resistant to every meaningful antibiotic that we had," Wetherbee recalled recently. The microbe was sensitive only to a drug called colistin, which had been developed decades earlier and largely abandoned as a systemic treatment, because it can severely damage the kidneys. "So we had this report, and I looked at it and said to myself, 'My God, this is an organism that basically we can't treat.'"

Klebsiella is in a class of bacteria called gram-negative, based on its failure to pick up the dye in a Gram's stain test. (Gram-positive organisms, which include *Streptococcus* and *Staphylococcus*, have a different cellular structure.) It inhabits both humans and animals and can survive in water and on inanimate objects. We can carry it on our skin and in our noses and throats, but it is most often found in our stool, and fecal contamination on the hands of caregivers is the most frequent source of infection among patients. Healthy people can harbor *Klebsiella* to no detrimental effect; those with debilitating conditions, like liver disease or severe diabetes, or those recovering from major surgery, are most likely to fall ill. The bacterium is oval in shape, resembling a TicTac, and has a thick, sugar-filled outer coat, which makes it difficult for white blood cells to engulf and destroy it. Fimbria—fine, hairlike extensions that enable *Klebsiella* to adhere to the lining of the throat, trachea, and bronchi—project from the bacteria's surface; the attached microbes can travel deep into our lungs, where they destroy the delicate alveoli, the air sacs that allow us to obtain oxygen. The resulting hemorrhage produces a blood-filled sputum, nicknamed "currant jelly." *Klebsiella* can also attach to the urinary tract and infect the kidneys. When the bacteria enter the bloodstream, they release a fatty substance known as an endotoxin, which injures the lining of the blood vessels and can cause fatal shock.

Tisch Hospital has four intensive-care units, all in the east wing on the fifteenth floor, and at the time of the outbreak there were thirty-two intensive-care beds. The I.C.U.s were built in 1961, and although the equipment had been modernized over the years, the units had otherwise remained relatively unchanged: the beds were close to each other, with I.V. pumps and respirators between them, and doctors and nursing staff were shared among the various I.C.U.s. This was an ideal environment for a highly infectious bacterium.

It was the first major outbreak of this multidrug-resistant strain of *Klebsiella* in the United States, and Wetherbee was concerned that the bacterium had become so well adapted in the I.C.U. that it could not be killed with the usual ammonia and phenol disinfectants. Only bleach seemed able to destroy it. Wetherbee and his team instructed doctors, nurses, and custodial staff to perform meticulous hand washing, and had them wear gowns and gloves when attending to infected patients. He instituted strict protocols to insure that gloves were changed and hands vigorously disinfected after handling the tubing on each patient's ventilator. Spray bottles with bleach solutions were installed in the I.C.U.s, and surfaces and equipment were cleaned several times a day. Nevertheless, in the ensuing months *Klebsiella* infected more than a dozen patients.

In late autumn of 2000, in addition to pneumonia patients began contracting urinary-tract and bloodstream infections from *Klebsiella*. The latter are often lethal, since once *Klebsiella* infects the bloodstream it can spread to every organ in the body. Wetherbee reviewed procedures in the I.C.U. again and discovered that the Foley catheters, used to drain urine from the bladder, had become a common source of contamination; when emptying the urine bags, staff members inadvertently splashed infected urine onto their gloves and onto nearby machinery. "They were very effectively moving the organism from one bed to the next," Wetherbee said. He ordered all the I.C.U.s to be decontaminated; the patients were temporarily moved out, supplies discarded, curtains changed, and each room was cleaned from floor to ceiling with a bleach solution. Even so, of the thirty-four patients with infections that year, nearly half died. The outbreak subsided in October, 2003, after even more stringent procedures for decontamination and hygiene were instituted: patients kept in isolation, and staff and visitors required to wear gloves, masks, and gowns at all times.

"My basic premise," Wetherbee said, "is that you take a capable microörganism like *Klebsiella* and you put it through the gruelling test of being exposed to a broad spectrum of antibiotics and it will eventually defeat your efforts, as this one did." Although Tisch Hospital has not had another outbreak, the bacteria appeared soon after at several hospitals in Brooklyn and one in Queens. When I spoke to infectious-disease experts this spring, I was told that the resistant *Klebsiella* had also appeared at Mt. Sinai Medical Center, in Manhattan, and in hospitals in New Jersey, Pennsylvania, Cleveland, and St. Louis.

Of the so-called superbugs—those bacteria that have developed immunity to a wide number of antibiotics—the methicillin-resistant *Staphylococcus aureus*, or MRSA, is the most well known. Dr. Robert Moellering, a professor at Harvard Medical School, a past president of the Infectious Diseases Society of America, and a leading expert on antibiotic resistance, pointed out that MRSA, like *Klebsiella*, originally occurred in I.C.U.s, especially among patients who had undergone major surgery. "Until about ten years ago," Moellering told me, "virtually all cases of MRSA were either in hospitals or nursing homes. In the hospital setting, they cause wound infections after surgery, pneumonias, and blood-stream infections from indwelling catheters. But they can cause a variety of other infections, all the way to bacterial meningitis." The first deaths from MRSA in community settings, reported at the end of the nineteen-nineties, were among children in North Dakota and Minnesota. "And then it started showing up in men who have sex with men," Moellering said. "Soon, it began to be spread in prisons among the prisoners. Now we see it in a whole bunch of other populations." An outbreak among the St. Louis Rams football team, passed on through shared equipment, particularly affected the team's linemen; artificial turf, which causes skin abrasions that are prone to infection, exacerbated the problem. Other outbreaks were reported among insular religious groups in rural New York; Hurricane Katrina evacuees; and illegal tattoo recipients. "And now it's basically everybody," Moellering said. The deadly toxin produced by the strain of MRSA found in U.S. communities, Panton-Valentine leukocidin, is thought to destroy the membranes of white blood cells, damaging the body's primary defense against the microbe. In 2006, the Centers for Disease Control and Prevention recorded some nineteen thousand deaths and a hundred and five thousand infections from MRSA.

Unlike resistant forms of *Klebsiella* and other gram-negative bacteria, however, MRSA can be treated. "There are about a dozen new antibiotics coming on the market in the next couple of years," Moellering noted. "But there are no good drugs coming along for these gram-negatives." *Klebsiella* and similarly classified bacteria, including *Acinetobacter*, *Enterobacter*, and *Pseudomonas*, have an extra cellular envelope that MRSA lacks, and that hampers the entry of large molecules like antibiotic drugs. "The *Klebsiella* that caused particular trouble in New York are spreading out," Moellering told me. "They have very high mortality rates. They are sort of the doomsday-scenario bugs."

In 1968, Moellering travelled to Malaita, in the Solomon Islands. "I was really interested to see whether we could find an antibiotic-resistant population of bacteria in a place that had never seen antibiotics," Moellering said. The natives practiced head-hunting and cannibalism, and were isolated as much by conflict as by the island's dense jungle. Moellering identified microbes there that were resistant to the antibiotics streptomycin and tetracycline, which were then in use in the West but had never been introduced clinically on Malaita. Later studies found resistant bacteria in many other isolated indigenous human populations, as well as in natural reservoirs like aquifers.

Before the development of antibiotics, the threat of infection was urgent: until 1936, pneumonia was the No. 1 cause of death in the United States, and amputation was sometimes the only cure for infected wounds. The introduction of sulfa drugs, in the nineteen-thirties, and penicillin, in the nineteen-forties, suddenly made many bacterial infections curable. As a result, doctors prescribed the drugs widely—often for sore throats, sinus congestion, and coughs that were due not to bacteria but to viruses. In response, bacteria quickly developed resistance to the most common antibiotics. The public assumed that the pharmaceutical industry and researchers in academic hospitals would continue to identify effective new treatments, and for many years they did. In the nineteen-eighties, a class of drugs called carbapenems was developed to combat gram-negative organisms like *Klebsiella*, *Pseudomonas*, and *Acinetobacter*. "They were, at the time, thought to be drugs of last resort, because they had activity against a whole variety of multiply-resistant gram-negative bacteria that were already floating around," Moellering said. Many hospitals put the drugs "on reserve," but an apparent cure-all was too tempting for some physicians, and the tight stewardship slowly broke down. Inevitably, mutant, resistant microbes flourished, and even the carbapenems' effectiveness waned.

Now microbes are appearing far outside their environmental niches. *Acinetobacter* thrives in warm, humid climates, like Honduras, as well as in parts of Iraq, and is normally found in soil. An article published in the military magazine *Proceedings* in February reported that more than two hundred and fifty patients at U.S. military hospitals were infected with a highly resistant strain of *Acinetobacter* between 2003 and 2005, with seven deaths as of June, 2006, linked to "*Acinetobacter*-related complications." In 2004, about thirty per cent of all patients returning from Iraq and Afghanistan tested positive for the bacteria. "It's a big problem, and it's contaminated the evacuation facilities in Germany and a lot of the V.A. hospitals in the United States where these soldiers have been brought," Moellering said. Patients evacuated to Stockholm from Thailand after the 2004 tsunami were often infected with resistant gram-negative microbes, including a strain of *Acinetobacter* that was resistant even to colistin, the antibiotic used, to variable effect, in the outbreak at Tisch Hospital. The practice of "clinical tourism," in which patients travel long distances for more advanced or more affordable medical centers, may introduce resistant microbes into hospitals where they had not existed before.

Meanwhile, antibiotic use in agricultural industries has grown rapidly. "Seventy per cent of the antibiotics administered

in America end up in agriculture," Michael Pollan, a professor of journalism at Berkeley and the author of "In Defense
of Food: An Eater's Manifesto," told me. "The drugs are not
used to cure sick animals but to prevent them from getting sick,
because we crowd them together under filthy circumstances.
These are perfect environments for disease. And we also have
found, for reasons that I don't think we entirely understand,
that administering low levels of antibiotics to animals speeds
their growth." The theory is that by killing intestinal bacteria the
competition for energy is reduced, so that the animal absorbs
more energy from the food and therefore grows faster. The Food
and Drug Administration, which is often criticized for its lack
of attention to the risks of widespread use of antibiotics, offers
recommended, non-binding guidelines for these drugs but has
rarely withdrawn approval for their application. A spokesman
for the Center for Veterinary Medicine at the F.D.A. told me
that the center "believes that prudent drug-use principles are
essential to the control of antimicrobial resistance." A study
by David L. Smith, Jonathan Dushoff, and J. Glenn Morris,
published by *PLoS Medicine*, from the *Public Library of Science*,
in 2005, noted that the transmission of resistant bacteria from
animal to human populations is difficult to measure, but that
"antibiotics and antibiotic-resistant bacteria (ARB) are found in
the air and soil around farms, in surface and ground water, in
wild-animal populations, and on retail meat and poultry. ARB
are carried into the kitchen on contaminated meat and poultry, where other foods are cross-contaminated because of common unsafe handling practices." The researchers developed
a mathematical model that suggested that the impact of the
transmission of these bacteria from agriculture may be more
significant than that of hospital transmissions. "The problem is
that we have created the perfect environment in which to breed
superbugs that are antibiotic-resistant," Pollan told me. "We've
created a petri dish in our factory farms for the evolution of
dangerous pathogens."

Ten years ago, the Institute of Medicine of the National Academy of Sciences, in Washington, D.C., assessed the economic impact of resistant microbes in the United States at up to five billion dollars, and experts now believe the figure to be much higher. In July, 2004, the Infectious Diseases Society of America released a white paper, "Bad Bugs, No Drugs: As Antibiotic Discovery Stagnates . . . A Public Health Crisis Brews," citing 2002 C.D.C. data showing that, of that year's estimated ninety thousand deaths annually in U.S. hospitals owing to bacterial infection, more than seventy per cent had been caused by organisms that were resistant to at least one of the drugs commonly used to treat them. Drawing on these data, collected mostly from hospitals in large urban areas which are affiliated with medical schools, the Centers for Disease Control and Prevention found more than a hundred thousand cases of gram-negative antibiotic-resistant bacteria. No precise numbers for all infections, including those outside hospitals, have been calculated, but the C.D.C. also reported that, among gram-negative hospital-acquired infections, about twenty per cent were resistant to state-of-the-art drugs.

In April, I visited Dr. Stuart Levy, at Tufts University School of Medicine. Levy is a researcher-physician who has made key discoveries about how bacteria become resistant to antibiotics. In addition to the natural cell envelope of *Klebsiella*, Levy outlined three primary changes in bacteria that make them resistant to antibiotics. Each change involves either a mutation in the bacterium's own DNA or the importation of mutated DNA from another. (Bacteria can exchange DNA in the form of plasmids, molecules that are shared by the microbes and allow them to survive inhibitory antibiotics.) First, the bacteria may acquire an enzyme that can either act like a pair of scissors, cutting the drug into an inactive form, or modify the drug's chemical structure, so that it is rendered impotent. Thirty years ago, Levy discovered a second change: pumps inside the bacteria that could spit out the antibiotic once it had passed through the cell wall. His first reports were met with profound skepticism, but now, Levy told me, "most people would say that efflux is the most common form of bacterial resistance to antibiotics." The third change involves mutations that alter the inner contents of the microbe, so that the antibiotic can no longer inactivate its target.

Global studies have shown how quickly these bacteria can develop and spread. "This has been a problem in Mediterranean Europe that started about ten years ago," Dr. Christian Giske told me. Giske is a clinical microbiologist at Karolinska University Hospital, in Stockholm, who, with researchers in Israel and Denmark, recently reported on the worldwide spread of resistant gram-negative bacteria. He continued, "It started to get really serious during the last five or six years and has become really dramatic in Greece." A decade ago, only a few microbes in Southern Europe had multidrug resistance; now some fifty to sixty per cent of hospital-acquired infections are resistant.

Giske and his colleagues found that infection with a resistant strain of *Pseudomonas* increased, twofold to fivefold, a patient's risk of dying, and increased about twofold the patient's hospital stay. Like other experts in the field, Giske's team was concerned about the lack of new antibiotics being developed to combat gram-negative bacteria. "There are now a growing number of reports of cases of infections caused by gram-negative organisms for which no adequate therapeutic options exist," Giske and his colleagues wrote. "This return to the preantibiotic era has become a reality in many parts of the world."

Doctors and researchers fear that these bacteria may become entrenched in hospitals, threatening any patient who has significant health issues. "Anytime you hear about some kid getting snatched, you want to find something in that story that will convince you that that family is different from yours," Dr. Louis Rice, an expert in antibiotic resistance at Louis Stokes Cleveland VA Medical Center, told me. "But the problem is that any of us could be an I.C.U. patient tomorrow. It's not easy to convey this to people if it's not immediately a threat. You don't want to think about it. But it's actually anybody who goes into a hospital. This is scary stuff." Rice mentioned that he had a mild sinusitis and was hoping it would not need to be treated, because taking an antibiotic could change the balance of microbes in his body and make it easier for him to contract a pathogenic organism while doing his rounds at the hospital.

Genetic elements in the bacteria that promote resistance may also move into other, more easily contracted bugs. Moellering pointed out that, while *Klebsiella* seems best adapted to hospital settings, and poses the greatest risk to patients, other gram-negative bacteria—specifically *E. coli*, which is a frequent cause of urinary-tract infection in otherwise healthy people—have recently picked up the genes from *Klebsiella* which promote resistance to antibiotics.

In the past, large pharmaceutical companies were the primary sources of antibiotic research. But many of these companies have abandoned the field. "Eli Lilly and Company developed the first cephalosporins," Moellering told me, referring to familiar drugs like Keflex. "They developed a huge number of important anti-microbial agents. They had incredible chemistry and incredible research facilities, and, unfortunately, they have completely pulled out of it now. After Squibb merged with Bristol-Myers, they closed their antibacterial program," he said, as did Abbott, which developed key agents in the past treatment of gram-negative bacteria. A recent assessment of progress in the field, from U.C.L.A., concluded, "FDA approval of new antibacterial agents decreased by 56 per cent over the past 20 years (1998-2002 vs. 1983-1987)," noting that, in the researchers' projection of future development only six of the five hundred and six drugs currently being developed were new antibacterial agents. Drug companies are looking for blockbuster therapies that must be taken daily for decades, drugs like Lipitor, for high cholesterol, or Zyprexa, for psychiatric disorders, used by millions of people and generating many billions of dollars each year. Antibiotics are used to treat infections, and are therefore prescribed only for days or weeks. (The exception is the use of antibiotics in livestock, which is both a profit-driver and a potential cause of antibiotic resistance.)

"Antibiotics are the only class of drugs where all the experts, as soon as you introduce them clinically, we go out and tell everyone to try to hold it in reserve," Rice pointed out. "If there is a new cardiology drug, every cardiologist out there is saying that everyone deserves to be on it." In February, Rice wrote an editorial in the *Journal of Infectious Diseases* criticizing the lack of support from the National Institutes of Health; without this support, he wrote, "the big picture did not receive the attention it deserved." Rice acknowledges that there are competing agendas. "As loud as my voice might be, there are louder voices screaming 'AIDS,' " he told me. "And there are congressmen screaming 'bioterrorism.' " Rice came up with the acronym ESKAPE bacteria—*Enterococcus faecium, Staphylococcus aureus, Klebsiella pneumoniae, Acinetobacter baumanni, Pseudomonas aeruginosa,* and the *Entero-bacter* species—as a way of communicating the threat these microbes pose, and the Infectious Diseases Society is lobbying Congress to pass the Strategies to Address Antimicrobial Resistance Act, which would earmark funding for research on ESKAPE microbes and also set up clinical trials on how to limit infection and antibiotic resistance. Rice has also proposed studies to determine the most effective use—at what dosage, and for how long—of antibiotics for common infections like bronchitis and sinusitis.

Dr. Anthony Fauci is the director of the National Institute of Allergy and Infectious Diseases, which chairs the federal interagency working group on microbial resistance. Fauci told me that the government is acutely aware of the severity of the problem. He pointed out that the N.I.H. recently issued a call for proposals to study optimal use of antibiotics for common bacterial infections. It has also funded so-called "coöperative agreements," including one on *Klebsiella*, to facilitate public-private partnerships where the basic research from the institute or from university laboratories can be combined with development by a pharmaceutical or a biotech company. Even so, the total funding for studying the resistance of ESKAPE microbes is about thirty-five million dollars, a fraction of the two hundred million dollars provided by the NIAID for research on antimicrobial resistance, most of which goes to malaria, t.b., and H.I.V. "The difficulty that we are faced with is that our budget has been flat for the last five years," Fauci told me. "In real dollars, we've lost almost fifteen per cent purchasing power," because of an inflation index of about three per cent for biomedical research and development.

Since September 11, 2001, significant funding has been directed toward the study of anthrax and other microbes, like the one that causes plague, which could be used as bioweapons. Although there is little concern that *Klebsiella* or *Acinetobacter* might be weaponized, the basic science of their mutation and resistance could be useful in helping us to understand these threats. Fauci hopes to make the case that funds for biodefense should be used to study the ESKAPE bugs, but, for now, he is quick to point out the challenge posed by a lack of resources. "The problem is, it is extremely difficult to do a prospective controlled trial, because when people come into the hospital they immediately get started on some treatment, which ruins the period of study," he said, referring to research into the treatment of common infections. "The culture of American medicine makes a study like that more difficult to execute."

These types of studies—on how often, and for how long, antibiotics should be prescribed—are much easier to conduct in countries where medicine is largely socialized and prescriptions are tightly regulated. Recently, researchers in Israel, where most citizens receive their care through such a system, showed that refraining from empirically prescribing antibiotics during the summer months resulted in a sharp decline in ear infections caused by antibiotic-resistant microbes. (In the United States, a 1998 study estimated that fifty-five per cent of all antibiotics prescribed for respiratory infections in outpatients—22.6 million prescriptions—were unnecessary.) In Sweden, the government closely monitors all infections, and has the power to intervene as needed. "Our infection-control people have a lot of authority," Giske said. "This is power from the legislation." Once a resistant microbe is identified, stringent protocols are put in place, with dramatic results. Fewer than two per cent of the *staphylococci* in Sweden are MRSA, compared with sixty per cent in the United States. "Of course, it's only around ten million people, so it's possible to intervene because everything is smaller," Giske said, adding, "Maybe Swedes are more used to this type of intervention and regulation."

Stuart Levy's laboratory occupies the eighth floor of a renovated building on Harrison Avenue in Boston's Chinatown, across the street from Tufts Medical Center. As I passed from his office into the corridor, I detected the acrid smell of agar, which is used to grow bacteria. That day, a laboratory technician was testing specimens taken from the eyes of people with bacterial conjunctivitis who had been given an antibiotic eye drop containing fluoroquinolone. Levy was comparing the bacteria from the infected eyes with those in the noses, cheeks, and throats of the same patients. His technician held up a petri dish with a cranberry-colored agar base. The patient's specimen was growing bacteria that were susceptible to the antibiotic; the drug had created a large oval clear zone on the plate which resembled the halo around the moon. The study investigates whether an antibiotic applied to the eye would affect bacteria in the nose and mouth as well, which might indicate that what seems to be an innocuous and limited treatment may profoundly change a wider area of the body and foster resistant microbes.

Levy has also received funding from the N.I.H. to study *Yersinia pestis*, the microbe that causes plague; the Department of Agriculture has sponsored his study of *Pseudomonas fluorescens*, a soil-based bacterium that has the potential to protect plants from microbial infection. He plans to develop it as a biocontrol agent, so that farmers can be weaned off the potent antibiotics and chemicals they use to treat their fields. "We need to treat biology with biology, not chemistry," he said. In other studies, Levy and his team are looking at ways to render bacteria nondestructive and noninvasive, so that they might enter the body without harmful effects. This makes it necessary to identify virulence factors—which parts of the bacteria cause damage to our tissues. Levy's laboratory is targeting a protein in gram-negative organisms called MAR, which appears to act as a master switch, turning on both virulence genes and genes that mediate resistance, like the efflux pump. In collaboration with a startup company called Paratek, of which Levy is a co-founder, his laboratory is screening novel compounds in the hope of finding a drug that blocks MAR.

Frederick Ausubel, a bacterial geneticist at the Massachusetts General Hospital, in Boston, is searching for drugs to combat bacterial virulence, using tiny animals like worms, which have intestinal cells that are similar to those in humans, and which are susceptible to lethal microbial infection. The worm that Ausubel is studying, *Caenorhabditis elegans*, is one and a half millimetres in length. "You are probably going to have to screen millions of compounds and you can't screen millions of infected mice," Ausubel said. "So our approach was to find an alternative host that could be infected with human pathogens which was small enough and cheap enough to be used in drug screens. What's remarkable is that many common human pathogens, including *Staphylococcus* and *Pseudomonas*, will cause intestinal infection and kill the worms. So now you can look for a compound that cures it, that prevents the pathogen from killing the host." Ausubel first screened some six thousand compounds by hand and found eight, none of them traditional antibiotics, that may protect the worms. He is also attempting, among other potential solutions, to find a compound that would block what is called "quorum sensing," in which bacteria release small molecules to communicate with one another and signal when a critical mass is present. Once this quorum is reached, the bacteria turn on their virulence genes. "Bacteria don't want to alert their host that they are there by immediately producing virulence factors which the host would recognize," triggering the immune system, Ausubel explained. "When they reach a certain quorum, there are too many of them for the host to do anything about it." Bonnie Bassler, a molecular biologist at Princeton University, has recently shown that it is through quorum sensing that cholera bacteria are able to accumulate in the intestines and release toxins that can be fatal; *Pseudomonas* is also known to switch on its virulence genes in response to signals from quorum sensing.

Moellering is enthusiastic but cautious about this avenue of research. "It's a great idea, but so far nobody has been able to make it work for human infections," he told me. With certain types of *staphylococci*, Moellering said, "mutations have occurred spontaneously in nature that cut down on a number of virulence factors . . . but they still cause serious infections. I'm not sure that we have a way yet to use what we know about virulence factors to develop effective antimicrobial agents. And we almost certainly will have to use these agents in combination with antibiotics." No one, Moellering said, has developed a way to disarm bacteria sufficiently to allow the human body to naturally and consistently defend against them. I asked him what we should do to combat these new superbugs. "Nobody has the answer right now," he said. "The fact of the matter is that we have found all the easy targets" for drug development. He went on, "So the only other thing we can do is continue to work on antibiotic stewardship." Meanwhile, new resistant bacteria, Moellering asserted, aren't going to go away. "We can temper things, we might be able to slow the rate of emergence of resistance, but it's unlikely that we will ever be able to conquer it."

Doctors Within Borders

Susanna Schrobsdorff

From *Newsweek*

What the massive turnout for a free medical and dental clinic in south-west Virginia reveals about the widening gap between health-care haves and have-nots in the United States.

SHEILA FOWLER IS 43. She has short brown hair, a soft, girlish voice and three grandchildren. What she does not have is teeth, or a way to pay for dentures. But Fowler is stoic; she jokes that she's got tough gums, adding that she can even eat pretzels if she sucks on them for a bit.

Fowler has made the hourlong journey from her home in Cleveland, Va., to the small town of Wise to take advantage of a huge annual medical and dental expedition set up by Remote Area Medical, a nonprofit organization that provides basic medical and dental care to people in the world's most inaccessible regions. This year, more than 1,800 volunteer doctors, dentists, nurses and assistants descended on the small town near the Kentucky border, setting up enormous field-hospital-style tents in which they saw roughly 2,500 patients over the course of two and a half days in late July. The Wise operation is coordinated locally by a team of nurses with the Health Wagon, a tiny health-care outreach program.

By the end of the weekend, the medical team, had extracted 3,857 painfully decayed teeth, administered 156 mammograms, screened hundreds of people for diabetes and heart disease, and given out 1,003 pairs of eyeglasses. About 30 people, chosen by lottery, were fitted for free dentures. Hundreds of people were turned away by volunteers who headed off cars at the main intersection when the clinic reached capacity.

RAM events such as the one in Wise—the Knoxville, Tenn.-based group runs about 15 similar clinics around the world every year, from Guyana to East Africa and rural parts of Appalachia—underscore the health-care dilemmas of the poorest Americans. Fowler's case is a prime example: She has almost no income after an auto accident left her unable to do her restaurant job. She's covered by the state Medicaid program, but Medicaid doesn't cover any preventive or routine dental care for adults. It will pay for emergency extractions, but, for Fowler, as for many others in areas where dentists are scarce, finding one that will take Medicaid payments isn't easy. That's why she came to Wise in 2003 to have her teeth pulled for free.

When she got her lower teeth out, volunteer dentists told Fowler that she had a few that could be saved, but she begged them to take every single one. "I said, 'Do it now while I'm here so that a week from now, after you're all gone, I don't have an infected tooth'," she remembers.

She has come back to Wise this year to see if she can get dentures and have some questions answered about diabetes, which she suffers from, along with arthritis from the auto accident. It's a hot Thursday evening, and the clinic, which is held at the county fairgrounds, won't open till the next morning. But Fowler, her 28-year-old daughter and her daughter's husband, both of whom say they also urgently need painful teeth pulled, are camping to be sure they get a good spot in line.

They aren't the only ones. By 8 P.M. on Thursday, the parking lot is jammed with people hoping to be among the lucky patients who make it in to see the volunteer medical staff. At least 200 are turned away. Those who have gotten there early enough have their numbered blue admission tickets in hand. They don't even flinch when they're told that they're in for yet another six-hour wait.

"We see people waiting in those long lines, and I simply don't know how they tolerate the pain they must be in because of infection and bleeding in their mouth," says Terry Dickinson, executive director of the Virginia Dental Association. And, says Dickinson, patients still are amazed that they don't have to pay for their care here: "I told a young lady here that we could remove her teeth, she was in her 20s, and she just started crying. 'You mean, I don't have to pay for that?' she asked."

Virginia's governor, Tim Kaine, visited this year's RAM expedition with five of his staff members on its first and busiest day and met patients like these as he worked the lines of people waiting for care. Later he said that he finds the event "both depressing and inspiring at the same time." Southwest Virginia's coal-mining region lags behind much of the rest of the country and the state in health care—residents have vastly higher rates of diabetes, obesity and lung disease and lower income levels than the rest of Virginia—but Kaine says that the need for more comprehensive care goes far beyond these rural communities, and his is not the only state facing the double bind of a tightening economy and increasing health-care costs.

Peter Cunningham, a researcher with the Center for Studying Health System Change in Washington, D.C., agrees: "Yes, in Appalachia, the need is extreme, but this isn't just an isolated problem. This is just where all our national health-care problems converge: high cost, lack of access. This is where the most number of people fall through the cracks." According to a recent study he coauthored, about 20 percent of all Americans reported not getting or delaying needed medical care in the previous 12 months, up from 14 percent in 2003.

Cunningham says that for Medicaid patients, including 29 million children, the dental benefit is really a "phantom" benefit because of the challenge of finding a dentist who will accept Medicaid's low reimbursement rates. The problem is worse in rural areas, where there are too few dentists to begin with.

Governor Kaine points to the fact that two thirds of the 46 million uninsured in the United States have jobs but can't afford health insurance. "This is a matter of political will," he says. "Other nations have a lower GDP than we do, and they've made a political decision that their people are going to have health coverage, but we keep deciding not to."

"We like to believe that everyone can get the care they need," says Diane Rowland, executive vice president of the Kaiser Family Foundation. "But people who are low-income, work hard and don't have coverage through a job have to make harsh economic choices about their health care. That might be to have a tooth pulled instead of getting a crown. Or to go without care at all."

Kaine has gotten funding to set up a small satellite program of the Virginia Commonwealth University Dental School in Wise to serve some of the community year-round. Other programs, such as Save the Children, are setting up nutrition, exercise and health-education programs in schools that they hope will help improve both dental and overall health.

The Virginia Dental Association's Dickinson says that education of the next generation is key in changing the culture in this part of Virginia, where knowledge about dental care and nutrition is poor. The dire dental situation among the low-income populations of southwest Virginia, and parts of Kentucky and West Virginia, is emblematic of the larger health-care crisis—the region has higher rates of tooth loss than almost anywhere in the United States. (Nationally, 108 million people don't have dental insurance.)

"The diet here, which is high in processed, sugary foods because they're cheaper, promotes decay. And when your teeth hurt, you aren't going to be eating salads," he says. "And now we know that there's a suggested link between all kinds of systemic diseases from diabetes to heart disease and oral cancer and the bacteria in the mouth. It's a cascading effect."

Sheila Fowler and her daughter bear out Dickinson's emphasis on education. Martha Hopkins, like her mother, believes teeth are mostly a source of trouble and pain. She wasn't able to have all her teeth removed this year but will come back again next year, she says. Her mom, who wasn't one of the lucky 30 to get dentures fitted, explains why she thinks spending money on your teeth is a bad idea: "I had to have fillings when I was a kid, and that's the worst thing you ever did to your teeth. I really believe that. I'd never have fillings put in my teeth if I knew what I know now. Because when those fillings fall out, stuff gets in there and rots those teeth, and then you have to get them pulled anyway. When they see it, they ought to pull it instead of fooling with it.

"For Dickinson, the philosophical battle will have to come another day. For now, he's thinking about all the patients he had to send home without care on Sunday, the last day of the RAM expedition: "I had to go to the stands, where there were hundreds of people still waiting, and say we could only take 20 more. They rushed me with questions and showed me their teeth. I said they'd have to come see us in October when we go to Grundy, Va.

"In the meantime, he believes many of the patients who were turned away will have to make due with visits to the E.R. for tooth pain, where they'll likely be given antibiotics and a pain pill and sent home. "That'll only calm it down for a couple of weeks. It'll come back," he says.

Thankfully, so will RAM.

How to Help

If you'd like to contribute to or volunteer with the Remote Area Medical Foundation go to their Web site.

To volunteer or contribute to The Health Wagon, whose small staff brings health care to the people of Appalachia all year round, and who will be helping some of this year's RAM patients get follow-up treatment for urgent conditions, go to their Web site.

And, to help with education, nutrition and physical activity programs that help impoverished children in rural communities throughout the United States, go the Save the Children U.S.A. Web site.

To help Mission of Mercy, a nonprofit organization that provides free dental care to underserved populations in Virginia and West Virginia, go to the Virginia Dental Association's Web site and scroll to the bottom of the page for donation and volunteering information.

We Fought Cancer . . . And Cancer Won

Sharon Begley

From *Newsweek*

After billions spent on research and decades of hit-or-miss treatments, it's time to rethink the war on cancer.

THERE IS A blueprint for writing about cancer, one that calls for an uplifting account of, say, a woman whose breast tumor was detected early by one of the mammograms she faithfully had and who remains alive and cancer-free decades later, or the story of a man whose cancer was eradicated by one of the new rock-star therapies that precisely target a molecule that spurs the growth of malignant cells. It invokes Lance Armstrong, who was diagnosed with testicular cancer in 1996 and, after surgery and chemotherapy beat it back, went on to seven straight victories in the Tour de France. It describes how scientists wrestled child-hood leukemia into near submission, turning it from a disease that killed 75 percent of the children it struck in the 1970s to one that 73 percent survive today.

But we are going to tell you instead about Robert Mayberry. In 2002 a routine physical found a lesion on his lung, which turned out to be cancer. Surgeons removed the malignancy, which had not spread, and told Mayberry he was cured. "That's how it works with lung cancer," says oncologist Edward Kim of the University of Texas M. D. Anderson Cancer Center in Houston, who treated Mayberry. "We take it out and say, 'You're all set, enjoy the rest of your life,' because really, what else can we do until it comes back?" Two years later it did. The cancerous cells in Mayberry's lung had metastasized to his brain—either after the surgery, since such operations rarely excise every single microscopic cancer cell, or long before, since in some cancers rogue cells break away from the primary tumor as soon as it forms and make their insidious way to distant organs. It's impossible to know. Radiation therapy shrank but did not eliminate the brain tumors. "With that level of metastasis," says Kim, "it's not about cure. It's about just controlling the disease." When new tumors showed up in Mayberry's bones, Kim prescribed Tarceva, one of the new targeted therapies that block a molecule called epidermal growth factor receptor (EGFR) that acts like the antenna from hell: it grabs growth-promoting signals out of the goop surrounding a cancer cell and uses them to stimulate proliferation. Within six months—it was now the autumn of 2005—the tumors receded, and Mayberry, who had been unable to walk when the cancer infiltrated his brainstem and bones, was playing golf again. "I have no idea why Tarceva worked on him," says Kim. "We've given the same drug to patients in the same boat, and had no luck." But the luck ran out. The cancer came back, spreading to Mayberry's bones and liver. He lost his battle last summer.

We tell you about Mayberry because his case sheds light on why cancer is on track to kill 565,650 people in the United States this year—more than 1,500 a day, equivalent to three jumbo jets crashing and killing everyone aboard 365 days a year. First, it shows the disconnect between the bench and the bedside, between what science has discovered about cancer and how doctors treat it. Biologists have known for at least two decades that it is the rare cancer that can be completely cured through surgery. Nevertheless, countless proud surgeons keep assuring countless anxious patients that they "got it all." In Mayberry's case, says Kim, "my gut feeling is that [cells from the original lung tumor] were smoldering in other places the whole time, at levels so low not even a whole-body scan would have revealed them." Yet after surgery and, for some cancers, radiation or chemotherapy, patients are still sent back into the world with no regimen to keep those smoldering cells from igniting into a full-blown metastatic cancer or recurrence of the original cancer. Mayberry's story also shows the limits of "targeted" cancer drugs such as Tarceva, products of the golden age of cancer genetics and molecular biology. As scientists have learned in just the few years since the drugs' introduction, cancer cells are like brilliant military tacticians: when their original route to proliferation and invasion is blocked, they switch to an alternate, marching cruelly through the body without resistance.

We also tell you about Mayberry because of something Boston oncologist (and cancer survivor) Therese Mulvey told us. She has seen real progress in her 19 years in practice, but the upbeat focus on cancer survivors, cancer breakthroughs and miracle drugs bothers her. "The metaphor of fighting cancer implies the possibility of winning," she said after seeing the last of that day's patients one afternoon. "But some people are just not going to be cured. We've made tremendous strides against some cancers, but on others we're stuck, and even our successes buy some people only a little more time before they die of cancer anyway." She pauses, musing on how the uplifting stories and statistics—death rates from female breast cancer have fallen steadily since 1990; fecal occult blood testing and colonoscopy have helped avert some 80,000 deaths from colorectal cancer since 1990—can send the wrong message. "With cancer," says Mulvey, "sometimes death is not optional."

Yet it was supposed to be. In 1971 President Richard Nixon declared war on cancer (though he never used that phrase) in his State of the Union speech, and signed the National Cancer Act to make the "conquest of cancer a national crusade." It was a bold goal, and without it we would have made even less progress. But the scientists and physicians whom Nixon sent into battle have come up short. Rather than being cured, cancer is poised to surpass cardiovascular disease and become America's leading killer. With a new administration taking office in January, and with the new group Stand Up to Cancer raising $100 million (and counting) through its telethon on ABC, CBS and NBC on Sept. 5, there is no better time to rethink the nation's war on cancer.

In 2008, cancer will take the lives of about 230,000 more Americans—69 percent more—than it did in 1971. Of course, since the population is older and 50 percent larger, that raw number is misleading. A fairer way to examine progress is to look at age-adjusted rates. Those statistics are hardly more encouraging. In 1975, the first year for which the National Cancer Institute has solid age-adjusted data, 199 of every 100,000 Americans died of cancer. That rate, mercifully, topped out at 215 in 1991. In 2005 the mortality rate fell to 184 per 100,000, seemingly a real improvement over 1975. But history provides some perspective. Between 1950 and 1967, age-adjusted death rates from cancer in women also fell, from 120 to 109 per 100,000, found an analysis by the American Cancer Society just after Nixon's speech. In percentage terms, the nation made more progress in keeping women, at least, from dying of cancer in those 17 years, when cancer research was little more than a cottage industry propelled by hunches and trial-and-error treatment, as it did in the 30 years starting in 1975, an era of phenomenal advances in molecular biology and genetics. Four decades into the war on cancer, conquest is not on the horizon. As a somber statement on the NCI Web site says, "the biology of the more than 100 types of cancers has proven far more complex than imagined at that time." Oncologists resort to a gallows-humor explanation: "One tumor," says Otis Brawley of the ACS, "is smarter than 100 brilliant cancer scientists."

The meager progress has not been for lack of trying. Since 1971, the federal government, private foundations and companies have spent roughly $200 billion on the quest for cures. That money has bought us an estimated 1.5 million scientific papers, containing an extraordinary amount of knowledge about the basic biology of cancer. It has also brought real progress on a number of fronts, not least the invention of drugs for nausea, bowel problems and other side effects of the disease or treatment. "These have reduced suffering and changed people's ability to live with cancer," says Mulvey. In fact, just a few months after Nixon's call to arms, Bernard Fisher of the University of Pittsburgh began studies that would show that a woman with breast cancer has just as good a chance of survival if she receives a mastectomy rather than have her breast, chest-wall muscles and underarm tissue cut out, the standard at the time. The new approach spared millions of women pain and disfigurement. In 1985, treatment improved again when Fisher showed that lumpectomy followed by radiation to kill lingering cells was just as effective for many women as mastectomy. It wasn't a cure, but it mattered. "One can wait for the home run," says Fisher, now 90, "but sometimes you get runs by hitting singles and doubles. We haven't hit a home run yet; we can't completely prevent or completely cure breast cancer."

Nixon didn't issue his call to arms in order to reduce disfigurement, however. The goal was "to find a cure for cancer." And on that score, there are some bright spots. From 1975 to 2005, death rates from breast cancer fell from 31 to 24 per 100,000 people, due to earlier detection as well as more-effective treatment. Mortality from colorectal cancer fell from 28 to 17 per 100,000 people, due to better chemotherapy and, even more, to screening: when colonoscopy finds precancerous polyps, they can be snipped out before they become malignant.

But progress has been wildly uneven. The death rate from lung cancer rose from 43 to 53 per 100,000 people from 1975 to 2005. The death rate from melanoma rose nearly 30 percent. Liver and bile-duct cancer? The death rate has almost doubled, from 2.8 to 5.3 per 100,000. Pancreatic cancer? Up from 10.7 to 10.8. Perhaps the most sobering statistic has nothing to do with cancer, but with the nation's leading killer, cardiovascular disease. Thanks to a decline in smoking, better ways to control hypertension and cholesterol and better acute care, its age-adjusted mortality has fallen 70 percent in the same period when the overall mortality rate from cancer has fallen 7.5 percent. No wonder cancer "is commonly viewed as, at best, minimally controlled by modern medicine, especially when compared with other major diseases," wrote Harold Varmus, former director of NCI and now president of Memorial Sloan-Kettering Cancer Center in New York, in 2006.

About all scientists knew about cancer 50 years ago was that cancer cells make copies of their DNA and then of themselves more rapidly than most normal cells do. In the 1940s, Sidney Farber, a Boston oncologist, intuited that since cells need a biochemical called folate to synthesize new DNA, an anti-folate might impede this synthesis. After a friend at a chemical company synthesized an anti-folate—it was named methotrexate—Farber gave it to cancer patients, sending some into short-term remission, he reported in 1948. (Two years earlier, scientists had serendipitously discovered that mustard gas, a chemical weapon, could reduce tumors in patients with non-Hodgkin's lymphoma, but no one had any idea how it worked.) Thus was born the era of chemotherapy, one that continues today. It is still based on the simple notion that disrupting DNA replication and cell division will halt cancer. Soon there would be dozens of chemo drugs that target one or more of the steps leading to cell proliferation. Almost all of those approved in the 1970s, 1980s and 1990s were the intellectual descendants of Farber's strategy of stopping cancer cells from making copies of their DNA, and then themselves, by throwing a biochemical wrench into any of the steps involved in those processes. And none of it had anything to do with understanding why cancer cells were demons of proliferation. "The clinical-research community was expending enormous effort mixing and matching chemotherapy drugs," recalls Dennis Slamon, who began a fellowship in oncology at UCLA in 1979 and is now director of clinical/translational research at the Jonsson Cancer Center there. "There was nothing coming out of the basic science that could help" patients.

In the high-powered labs funded by the war on cancer, molecular biologists thought they could change that. By discovering how genetic and other changes let cancer cells multiply like frisky rabbits, they reasoned, they could find ways to stop the revved-up replication at its source. That promised to be more effective, and easier on healthy cells than chemotherapy drugs, which also kill normal dividing cells, notably in the gut, bone marrow, mouth and hair follicles. In the 1970s, cancer scientists discovered cancer viruses that alter DNA in animals, and for a while the idea that viruses cause cancer in people, too, was all the rage. (The human papilloma virus causes cervical cancer, but other human cancers have nothing to do with viruses, it would turn out.) In the 1970s and 1980s they discovered human genes that, when mutated, trigger or promote cancer, as well as tumor suppressor genes that, when healthy, do as their name implies but when damaged release the brakes on pathways leading to cancer.

It made for a lot of elegant science and important research papers. But it "all seemed to have little or no impact on the methods used by clinicians to diagnose and treat cancers," wrote Varmus. Basic-science studies of the mechanisms leading to cancer and efforts to control cancer, he observed, "often seemed to inhabit separate worlds." Indeed, it is possible (and common) for cancer researchers to achieve extraordinary acclaim and success, measured by grants, awards, professorships and papers in leading journals, without ever helping a single patient gain a single extra day of life. There is no pressure within science to make that happen. It is no coincidence that the ratio of useful therapy per basic discovery is abysmal. For other diseases, about 20 percent of new compounds arising from basic biological discoveries are eventually approved as new drugs by the FDA. For cancer, only 8 percent are.

A widely discussed 2004 article in Fortune magazine ("Why We're Losing the War on Cancer") laid the blame for this at the little pawed feet of lab mice and rats, and indeed there is a lot to criticize about animal studies. The basic approach, beginning in the 1970s, was to grow human cancer cells in a lab dish, transplant them into a mouse whose immune system had been tweaked to not reject them, throw experimental drugs at them and see what happened. Unfortunately, few of the successes in mice are relevant to people. "Animals don't reflect the reality of cancer in humans," says Fran Visco, who was diagnosed with breast cancer in 1987 and four years later founded the National Breast Cancer Coalition, an advocacy group. "We cure cancer in animals all the time, but not in people." Even scientists who have used animal models to make signal contributions to cancer treatment agree. "Far more than anything else," says Robert Weinberg of MIT, the lack of good animal models "has become the rate-limiting step in cancer research."

For this story, NEWSWEEK combed through three decades of high-profile successes in mice for clues to why the mice lived and the people died. Two examples make the point. Scientists were tremendously excited when Weinberg and colleagues discovered the first cancer-causing gene (called ras) in humans, in 1982. It seemed obvious that preventing ras from functioning should roll back cancer. In this decade, scientists therefore began testing drugs, called FTIs, that do exactly that. When FTIs were tested on human cancers that had been implanted into mice, they beat back the cancer. But in people, the drugs failed. One reason, scientists suspect, is that the transplanted cancers came from tumors that had been growing in lab dishes for years, long enough to accumulate countless malignant genes in addition to ras. Disabling ras but leaving those other mutations free to stoke proliferation was like using a sniper to pick off one soldier in an invading platoon: the rest of the platoon marches on. That general principle—not even the malignancy in a single cancer has one cause—would haunt cancer research and treatment for years. A compound called TNF, for tumor necrosis factor, raised hopes in the 1980s that it would live up to its name. When it was injected into mice carrying human tumors, it seemed to melt them away. But in clinical trials, it had little effect on the cancer. "Animal models have not been very predictive of how well drugs would do in people," says oncologist Paul Bunn, who leads the International Society for the Study of Lung Cancer. "We put a human tumor under the mouse's skin, and that microenvironment doesn't reflect a person's—the blood vessels, inflammatory cells or cells of the immune system," all of which affect prognosis and survival.

If mouse models have a single Achilles' heel, it is that the human tumors that scientists transplant into them, and then attack with their weapon du jour, almost never metastasize. Even in the 1970s there was clear evidence—in people—of the deadly role played by cells that break off from the original tumor: women given chemo to mop up any invisible malignant cells left behind after breast surgery survived longer without the cancer's showing up in their bones or other organs, and longer, period, than women who did not receive such "adjuvant" therapy, scientists reported in 1975. "Every study of adjuvant therapy shows it works because it kills metastatic cells even when it appears the tumor is only in the breast or in the first level of lymph nodes," says the ACS's Brawley. By the mid-1990s studies had shown similar results for colon cancer: even when surgeons said they'd "got it all," patients who received chemo lived longer and their cancer did not return for more years.

Yet for years, despite the clear threat posed by metastatic cells, which we now know are responsible for 90 percent of all cancer deaths, the war on cancer ignored them. Scientists continued to rely on animal models where metastasis didn't even occur. Throughout the 1980s and 1990s, says Visco, "researchers drilled down deeper and deeper into the disease," looking for ever-more-detailed molecular mechanisms behind the initiation of cancer, "instead of looking up and asking really big questions, like why cancer metastasizes, which might help patients sooner."

There was another way. At the same time that molecular biologists were taking the glamorous, "look for the cool molecular pathway," *cojones*-fueled approach to seeking a cure, pediatric oncologists took a different path. Pediatric cancer had long been a death sentence: in Farber's day, children with leukemia rarely survived more than three months. (President Bush's sister Robin died of the disease in 1953; she was 3.) Fast-forward to 2008: 80 percent of children with cancer survive well into adulthood.

To achieve that success, pediatric oncologists collaborated to such a degree that at times 80 percent of the children with a particular cancer were enrolled in a clinical trial testing a new therapy. In adults, it has long been less than 1 percent. The researchers focused hardly at all on discovering new molecular pathways and new drugs. Instead, they threw everything into the existing medicine chest at the problem, tinkering with drug doses and combinations and sequencing and timing. "We were learning how to better use the drugs we had," says pediatric oncologist Lisa Diller of Dana-Farber Cancer Institute and Children's Hospital Boston. By 1994, combinations of four drugs kept 75 percent of childhood leukemia patients—and 95 percent of those enrolled in a study—cancer-free. Childhood brain cancer has been harder to tame, but while 10 percent of kids survived it in the 1970s, today 45 percent do—a greater improvement than in most adult cancers. (To be sure, some scientists who work on adult cancers are sick of hearing about the noble cooperation of their pediatric colleagues. Childhood cancers, especially leukemias, are simpler cancers, they say, often characterized by a single mutation, and that's why the cure rate has soared. Neutral observers say it's a little of both: pediatric-cancer scientists really did approach the problem in a novel, practical way, but their enemy is less wily than most adult cancers.)

Biologists who never met a signaling pathway they didn't love tend to dismiss the success in pediatric oncology. It involved no discoveries of elegant cell biology, just plodding work. Ironically, however, it is these "singles," not the grand slams of molecular biology, that have made the greatest difference in whether people develop cancer and die of it. Fewer smokers (54 percent of men smoked in 1971; 21 percent do today), more women having mammograms and fewer taking hormone-replacement therapy (the incidence of breast cancer fell an unheard-of 7 percent from 2002 to 2003, after a 2002 study found that HRT can stimulate the growth of tiny breast tumors) have had at least as great an impact on cancer as the achievements of basic-science labs that received the bulk of the funding in the war on cancer. Similarly, the widespread use of Pap smears to detect precancerous changes in cells of the cervix is almost entirely responsible for the drop in both incidence of and deaths from cervical cancer. Incidence has fallen some 65 percent since 1975, and mortality at least 60 percent. Little wonder, then, that by the 1980s critics were asking why the war on cancer was spending the vast majority of taxpayers' money on elegant biology that cured millions of mice rather than on the search for more practical advances like these.

By "critics," we don't mean disgruntled laypeople. At UCLA, Denny Slamon had been inspired by Robert Weinberg's discovery of the first human oncogene, ras, in 1982. Although drugs to squelch the gene directly did not pan out, the discovery did lead to the first real success of the reductionist, "let's get in there and study the genetics and molecules of cancer" approach. Slamon was at first following the crowd, examining animal cancers for signs of DNA changes. But in 1982 he had an idea: look for unusual genes in tissue samples taken from human tumors. He applied to NCI for funding and, he recalls, "they basically sent it back with a laugh track. They said it was just a fishing expedition, that it wasn't hypothesis-driven. We tried to explain the logic—that if cancer reflects a problem of genetic control, then finding mutated genes should be important—but still didn't get funded." The same year that NCI laughed at Slamon's idea, MIT's Weinberg and colleagues discovered another gene involved in cancer. Called HER2, it makes a molecule that sits on the outside of cells and acts like an antenna, picking up growth signals that are then carried to the cell nucleus, where they deliver a simple if insidious message: go forth and multiply, really really fast. That made Slamon wonder whether HER2 might play a role in major human cancers.

In 1984, backed by private funding, Slamon found that 27 percent of breast cancers contain extra copies of HER2. Over the next decade he and other scientists showed that HER2 caused the cancer, rather than being an innocent bystander (or "marker," as scientists say). They also found an antibody that attaches to HER2 like a squirrel's nest on a TV antenna, preventing it from picking up signals. In 1998 the FDA approved that antibody, called Herceptin, for use in breast cancers fueled by HER2. It was stunning proof of the principle that drugs could be precisely crafted to cripple molecules that lie upstream of cell replication, stoking the growth of cancer cells and only cancer cells, not healthy ones, and has cured thousands of women. After the 1984 discovery, NCI was happy to fund Slamon. "It was only because we had already shown that the research would work," he says wistfully. "It is, shall we say, a conservative way to spend your money."

Slamon was not the only scientist who noticed NCI's preference for elegant molecular studies over research that offered the possibility of new treatments. (We should note that funding decisions are made not by NCI bureaucrats but by panels of scientists from, mostly, universities and medical institutions.) In the mid-1990s Brain Druker of the Oregon Health and Science

University Cancer Institute wanted to study a molecule involved in chronic myelogenous leukemia. Targeting that molecule, he thought, might cure CML. "People rolled their eyes and asked, 'What's new and different about this?' " By "new and different," they meant scientifically novel, elegant, offering new insight into a basic cellular process. He didn't even apply for an NCI grant. "I knew I'd just be wasting my time," he says. "NCI would have looked at what I wanted to do and said it was too high-risk. Instead I took the tried-and-true approach of getting funded for basic research, seeing how cell growth is regulated" by molecules that are grabbed by receptors on a leukemia cell and that send proliferation orders to the cell nucleus. This work led to a useful clinical test, but the work NCI did not fund (a private foundation did) eventually led to Gleevec, the blockbuster CML drug.

Indeed, there is no more common refrain among critics of how the war on cancer has been waged: that innovative ideas, ideas that might be grand slams but carry the risk of striking out, are rejected by NCI in favor of projects that promise singles. "We ask the scientists all the time why aren't we further along," says Visco. "Part of the answer is that the infrastructure of cancer is to keep things moving along as they have been and to reward people doing safe research. Exciting new ideas haven't fared well." As coincidence would have it, in the very year that Nixon launched the war on cancer, an unknown biologist named Judah Folkman published a paper proposing that metastatic cells survive, and become deadly, only if they grow blood vessels to keep themselves supplied with nutrients. That process is called angiogenesis, and it had nothing to do with the genes and proteins that the soldiers in the war on cancer were fixated on. Throughout the 1970s "the reaction was mainly hostility and ridicule," Folkman (who died earlier this year) recalled to NEWSWEEK in 1998. "People would ask me [at scientific meetings], 'You really don't believe that, do you?' " NCI turned down his request for funds to continue his work, calling his ideas about the importance of angiogenesis in metastasis "just your imagination," Folkman said. He persisted, of course, laying the groundwork for what would become anti angiogenesis drugs. Avastin was approved for colorectal cancer in 2004.

If the 1990s were the era of identifying cellular processes and molecules unique to cancer cells—not the blunderbuss approach of wrecking DNA and stopping replication, which brings friendly fire down on healthy cells—the focus of the 2000s is to personalize treatment. The reason is that, just as cancer cells develop resistance to standard chemo drugs, so they are finding ways to elude the new targeted drugs such as Avastin, Gleevec and Herceptin. In the studies that led the FDA to approve Avastin, for instance, the drug prolonged life in patients with advanced colorectal cancer by a median of four months. In later studies, it increased survival in advanced lung-cancer patients by a couple of months, says Roy Herbst, a lung oncologist at M. D. Anderson. Why so little? "Angiogenesis is a redundant process," Herbst explains. "Most cells use the VEGF pathway [that Avastin blocks], but there are at least 12 other pathways, and Avastin doesn't block any of them." With VEGF out of commission, malignant cells turn to these alternatives. Or consider Tarceva, given to lung-cancer patients, which turns off a molecule called EGFR that fuels the proliferation of some lung and other cancer cells. "It shrinks the tumor 60 to 80 percent of the time, and the effect lasts about a year," says David Johnson, a thoracic oncologist at Vanderbilt (University) Ingram Cancer Center. But if even a tiny fraction of malignant cells in the tumor or at metastatic sites use a proliferation pathway other than EGFR, they laugh off Tarceva and proliferate unchecked; most patients are dead within three years. Of the first patients with a rare gastric cancer whom George Demetri of Dana-Farber treated with Gleevec in 2000, 85 percent became resistant to it after five years. (Before Gleevec, though, patients with this cancer died within six weeks.) The malignant cells, it turns out, change the shape of the molecule that Gleevec blocks. It's as if a teenager, knowing Mom has a key to his room and wanting his privacy, changed the lock before she arrived.

In response to the limits of targeted therapies, scientists are pursuing the next big idea: that there is no such thing as cancer. There are only cancers, plural, each one characterized by a different set of mutations, a different arsenal it uses to fight off drugs and proliferate. "By the time there are 10 cancer cells, you probably have eight different cancers," says Demetri. "There are different pathways in each of the cells." And that's why cancer patients keep dying. One woman found a lump in her breast in 2002, nine months after a mammogram had shown nothing amiss. She had the breast tumor removed, says oncologist Julie Gralow, who treated her at the Fred Hutchinson Cancer Center, and chemotherapy to kill any remaining malignant cells. The woman did well for three years, but in 2005 an exam found cancer in her bones. She underwent half a dozen different chemotherapies over the next three years, until last March the cancer was detected in her brain. She received radiation—because chemo drugs generally do not cross the blood-brain barrier, radiation rather than chemo is the treatment of choice for brain cancer—but by July tumors had riddled her body. She died that month.

To beat down cancer mortality, oncologists need to target all the many cancers that make up a cancer—the dozens of different pathways that cells use to proliferate and spread. That is the leading edge of research today, determining how *this* patient's tumor cells work and hitting those pathways with multiple drugs, simultaneously or sequentially, each chosen because it targets one of those growth, replication and angiogenesis pathways. "The hope is to match tumor type to drug," says Roy Herbst. "We need to make the next leap, getting the right drug to the right patient."

Both presidential candidates have vowed to support cancer research, which makes this a propitious time to consider the missed opportunities of the first 37 years of the war on cancer.

Surely the greatest is prevention. Nixon never used the word; he exhorted scientists only to find a cure. Partly as a result, the huge majority of funding for cancer has gone into the search for ways to eradicate malignant cells rather than to keep normal cells from becoming malignant in the first place. "The funding people are interested in the magic-bullet research because that's what brings the dollars in," says oncologist Anthony Back, of the Hutch. "It's not as sexy to look at whether broccoli sprouts prevent colon cancer. A reviewer looks at that and asks, 'How would you ever get that to work?' " And besides, broccoli can't be patented, so without the potential payoff of a billion-dollar drug there is less incentive to discover how cancer can be prevented.

Another missed opportunity involves the environment around a tumor cell. "We used to focus on cancer cells with the idea that they were master of their own destiny," says MIT's Weinberg. "By studying genes inside the cell we thought we could understand what was going on. But now [we know] that many tumors are governed by the signals they receive from outside"— from inflammatory cells, cells of the immune system and others. "It's the interaction of signals inside and outside the tumor that creates aggressiveness and metastasis."

Which leads to the third big missed opportunity, the use of natural compounds and nondrug interventions such as stress reduction to keep the microenvironment inhospitable to cancer. (Cancer cells have receptors that grab stress hormones out of the bloodstream and use them to increase angiogenesis.) "Funding has gone to easier areas to research, like whether a drug can prevent cancer recurrence," says Lorenzo Cohen, who runs the integrative care center at M. D. Anderson. That's simpler to study, he points out, than whether a complicated mix of diet, exercise and stress reduction techniques can keep the microenvironment hostile to cancer. And while we're on the subject of how to reduce mortality from cancer, consider these numbers: 7 percent of black women with breast cancer get no treatment, 35 percent do not receive radiation after mastectomy (the standard of care), and 26 percent of white women do not. As long as scientists are discovering how to thwart cancer, it might make sense to get the advances into the real world.

Breakthroughs continue to pour out of labs, of course. Cutting-edge techniques are allowing scientists to identify promising experimental drugs more quickly than ever before. And just last week separate groups of scientists announced that they had identified dozens of genes involved in glioblastoma, the most common brain cancer, as well as pancreatic cancer. That raises the possibility that the mutations cause the cancer, and that if the pathways they control can be blocked the cancer can be beaten back. Stop us if you've heard that before. Hope springs eternal that such findings will not join the long list of those that are interesting but irrelevant to patients.

Duality

Julie R. Rosenbaum

from *Health Affairs*

In the late twentieth century, as more and more women entered the medical profession and became mothers, people wondered what it would mean. As might have been expected, there are many realities. For Julie Rosenbaum, who teaches in a primary care internal residency program, a major concern is how she and her husband juggle their jobs with raising young children. In a split-voice narrative, Rosenbaum details the dual focus of her days and how they interact. As she and her husband ponder what's best, she reports that academic medicine is simultaneously pondering how best to work with and support doctor-parents. Then pediatrician and professor Anjali Jain tells what happened when her family moved from the U.S. to the U.K. and her special-needs child wasn't well diagnosed or cared for by England's National Health Service. As a doctor, she knew there was a problem; as a mother, she did all she could to find a solution. Eventually, she and her husband made a choice and found a solution—an American one.

MORNING: AS USUAL, I didn't get enough sleep last night. The alarm goes off at 6 A.M.; I hear the baby stirring. I'm alone in bed. My husband left early to take the train into the city, where he works as an academic scientist. Today I'll take the children to and from day care. Despite my multiple responsibilities at home and the office, each work day is bounded by the transitions where I transfer my children to and from the care of others. Even on days when my husband helps, which he does several times a week, I still attend to many of the details. Each transfer is a carefully orchestrated event where each detail must be addressed, from each piece of clothing to every morsel of food. Any deviation from the norm can throw the entire process and day's productivity out of whack. At work I pace myself carefully, with close attention to the clock. If I leave the office late, I'll be late to pick up the children, owe the day care center additional money, and bear the weight of substantial guilt and, perhaps, tears.

I entered medicine at a time when opportunities for women in the profession were soaring. As of 2004, more than 50 percent of entering students were women.[1] But despite increasing numbers of women at lower ranks in academia, as in other fields, fewer women have achieved the highest echelon, including full professorships (16 percent), department chairs (10 percent), or medical school deans (11 percent). In fact, given the number of women entering medicine, the accomplishments at these levels are lower than would be expected.[2] The reasons proposed for this discrepancy are many, including a glass ceiling caused by a lack of mentors, unsupportive environments, lack of flexible academic pathways, inadequate promotion and retention, and frank sexism.[3] Of note: Women are also still paid less for the same work, even when adjustments are made for years of training, career publications, department type, and hours worked.[4] Some have suggested that part of the gender discrepancy—in terms of achieving the highest academic posts—is because women choose to forgo professional opportunities as a trade-off for their parental obligations and pleasures.[5]

My three-year-old daughter, the baby, and I make it downstairs to the kitchen. Peeking at the clock, I prepare for the morning ritual. Today is Monday, always the worst day of the week, because in addition to everything else, I have to get the bedding bags to day care. One backpack per child, each including a blanket, sheets, a stuffed animal, and strategic changes of clothes, packed last night. The coffee is made; now I focus on the baby's nourishment for the day. I fill four bottles with breast milk that I pumped last month, stored in the freezer, and defrosted overnight. Don't forget the ice pack! Then I prepare the materials for the breast pump to take to work today. For this I have to unload the dishwasher. I need the breast shields, the four milk receptacles, and a fresh cloth for the handy-dandy, super stylish, and very subtle breast pump backpack. Can't forget the ice pack! I know I could make my life easier by stopping breastfeeding at this point—the baby's seven months old—but it's not a compromise I'm willing to make.

The baby starts to cry. I pick him up and do my usual comfort routine, but he seems less consolable than normal, although not hot. I hope this isn't the beginning of something. My mind races. What if the baby's sick and can't go to day care? My husband's already gone. My college-student babysitter has class today. My mother-in-law's traveling. Perhaps this crankiness is nothing, and I can still make my faculty meeting and clinical responsibilities. Suddenly, I realize that my daughter isn't at the table eating; this might throw off everything. I call her for breakfast. Where was I? My daughter's lunch. My husband had prepared it the night before, and it's in the fridge. Don't forget the ice pack! I need to go the supermarket, but time's the problem. I should be reading my pile of medical journals. I should be working on that manuscript I started before the baby was born. I should. I should . . .

To redress the gender imbalance in academic medicine, several initiatives have been developed. These include mentoring networks, flexible career paths, and more robust parental leave policies. I benefit from an institution that takes part-time work seriously, allowing my progression on my academic clock to be prorated and where I received an additional year in my current term when I had my baby.

Some of these policies, however, have had unanticipated consequences that, instead of leveling the playing field, have led to unexpected results. For example, some departments in other academic institutions made semester-long parental leaves available to both genders. Despite the just intention of these policies, reports emerged of men using these periods as if they were sabbaticals; they left the primary child care to their wives and used the freed-up time to further their publication records.[6] A policy at Harvard Law School, which provides for parental leave with an explicit expectation of the parent providing at least twenty hours of primary child care during daytime and weekday hours, seeks to redress such abuses.

Now the baby's clearly unhappy. I remove his diaper to check a rectal temperature and find a foul diaper and a raging diaper rash. I verify that there's no fever, and he fights me terribly as I apply diaper cream. I pick him up again, and he is sobbing uncontrollably. Is this just diaper rash or something else brewing? Is it safe to bring him to day care? Is there a communicable infection at play? What would I say to my coworkers? "My son's diaper rash was out of control; you have to cover my teaching responsibilities this afternoon. Sorry!"

I know many people who'd just give him ibuprofen at moments like these, bring him to day care, and hope for the best. My son continues to cry miserably and not let me put him down. I just can't do this. What are my priorities, anyway? My daughter comes over and hugs me when she sees how upset I am. It's an embrace like this that reminds you how unbelievably incredible it is to be a parent.

Regardless of my proposed plans for the day, the baby needs some pain reliever; thankfully, he takes the ibuprofen easily. I sway with him as I eat my cereal standing up, giving a final warning to my daughter that it's time to finish getting dressed and go to the bathroom before we leave. The baby starts to settle, and I again focus on departure.

Beyond parental leave, further research has discovered additional aspects of the faculty/parenting challenge. Women with children have less successful academic progress than their male colleagues or women without children.[7] Another qualitative study corroborating this finding quotes a female department chair who notes that women who have successful family lives do not seem as likely to ascend to certain levels in academia, that all women who have reached the higher echelon are "divorced or lesbians."[8] In fact, an experiment involving volunteers pretending to be employers making decisions about hiring found that mothers, as opposed to fathers or female nonmothers, were believed to be less competent and committed and received job offers less often.[9] When they did receive offers, the salary rate was significantly lower than for nonmother applicants. They were also deemed less likely to be promoted.

We go to the living room, and I itemize. The baby's bedding bag and bottle bag. My daughter's bedding bag and lunch box. My computer bag and briefcase. My breast pump. This is ridiculous. We're all dressed. I take the bags and baby to the car in two trips. With strange mix of relief and apprehension, I note that the baby is falling asleep as I secure him into the car seat. With both children strapped in, we're ready to go.

By the time I drop the children off, set up their things for the day, and commute to work, I've been up for about three hours. I'm absolutely exhausted and just want to take a nap. Finally, I take my seat at the faculty meeting.

Afternoon: I enter the room with the intern at 4 p.m. He's already presented his assessment of the patient's situation to me, and I want to be present when he discusses our plan with her. I know that I must keep my eye on the clock and be walking to the parking lot by 4:15 p.m. My son's done well at day care; the irritability was just a terrible diaper rash after all. I've attended to my responsibilities today, despite a slightly higher level of distraction than normal. After my departure, my colleagues will help the residents finish their patients, and I will pay them back on other days.

The patient is a young woman who's had four children by age twenty-three. She tries to run a hair salon out of her home. She is currently estranged from her significant other, who is not the father of any of the children. She has little family nearby and somehow pulls together help from friends to watch her daughters at key moments of her day. The intern's assessed the young woman for fatigue and is concerned about her inability to sleep.

He tells her that we'll check her blood count and thyroid to eliminate certain physical explanations for her fatigue, but that we are concerned that she is depressed. Suddenly, a tear falls from her eye. She says she feels sad and stressed but that she believes depression is a sign of weakness. She won't be open to trying medication as she thinks her family wouldn't approve; she can't be seen as having a mental illness. The intern looks to me with a fraught expression.

I glance subtly at the clock. I only have a few minutes left. My options are to call the college student back-up babysitter or call in my faculty colleague to help the intern—but by the time I explain the situation, I might as well handle it myself. I might not be able to give the patient the explanation, time, or comfort that I think she deserves. Or my daughter will make me feel guilty for being late. Plus, the kids have already had such a long day in day care. So much for respect for the primacy of patient welfare, one of the fundamental tenets of the medical profession.

I sit with the patient, holding her hand. We review some other options, including counseling and support groups; each seems impractical given the daily demands on her life. We confirm that she isn't suicidal. We reassure her that we'll work with her and try to help her get to a better place. I ask her to return in two weeks to review the lab results and see how she is doing. "I am just trying to do the best I can . . . " she says. I look her in the eye and say, "I know, I know . . ." Physicians are supposed to try to understand our patients' perspectives as if we were standing in their shoes. Despite my daily challenges, I could never fully appreciate her struggle to care for herself and her children. As harried as I sometimes feel, I count my blessings and appreciate the resources and opportunity I have.

According to an analysis of the work of the average U.S. mother, if you consider each component of a mother's role (for example, housekeeper, cook, launderer, van driver, and psychologist), she would earn $134,121 a year in salary.[10] The immutable work of the home still takes time and effort, and it doesn't go away when both parents work. According to the U.S. Department of Labor, even in dual-income households, women continue to take greater responsibility for housework and child care than do men, spending close to an hour and a half more each day caring for their home and family and an hour less at work.[11]

The intern and I step out and quickly confirm the plan, and I grab my coat, computer bag, briefcase, and breast pump, wave to my colleague, and clumsily scamper out. Sometimes I feel compromised on all sides, as a parent, teacher, physician, and person. Once on the road, I give a hands-free call to the intern to talk about one more social work alternative for the patient. I watch the speedometer.

Given the stresses of the day, I again contemplate if my husband and I have arranged our situation appropriately. I'm often overwhelmed with how much mental and emotional energy this topic consumes. Having a nanny would make the start and end of the day easier. But it would be substantially more expensive and subject our children and our work lives to major disruption if she quits, as we learned the hard way. And if we got more help, would I feel guilty spending less time with my kids? Maybe.

It's time to take more advantage of the college students in town for babysitting help, to find a nice, responsible kid with a car. Even with this option, however, we'll have to work around vacations, finals, and health issues. No solution is perfect, and redundancy in the system is crucial. Each family works out its own balance and, importantly, makes adjustments each year as children progress through school. I'm almost paralyzed when I contemplate how to arrange my schedule once my children grow and have more activities that I'll want to encourage and attend. Take a deep breath. Take it one year at a time. Take it one day at a time.

Many women have given up on the notion that they can have it all, at least at the same time.[12] We desire flexibility and alternative pathways, but also not to be discounted or undervalued simply because we are also mothers. We hope that our husbands can continue to contribute to more of the household activities through increasing job flexibility—as do they.[13] Increasing fathers' ability and time to be involved in their families might help our children's academic achievement and social development.[14] These changes, however, can be achieved only through leadership and workplace policies that create environments allowing men and women to be involved in their families without the weight of cultural biases that might hinder any parent from reaching his or her full potential, either as a professional or as a parent.

Luckily, traffic is moving well this evening. I should be at the day care center almost on time. My children will likely be alone with the teachers; I'll give each child a huge hug.

1. D. Magrane and P. Lange, "An Overview of Women in U.S. Academic Medicine, 2005–2006," Analysis in Brief 6, no. 7 (2006): 1–2.
2. A.S. Ash et al., "Compensation and Advancement of Women in Academic Medicine: Is There Equity?" Annals of Internal Medicine 141, no. 3 (2004): 205–212; and L. Nonnemaker, "Women Physicians in Academic Medicine: New Insights from Cohort Studies," New England Journal of Medicine 342, no. 6 (2000): 399–405.
3. J. Bickel et al., "Increasing Women's Leadership in Academic Medicine: Report of the AAMC Project Implementation Committee," Academic Medicine 77, no. 10 (2002): 1043–1061; and M.J. Yedidia and J. Bickel, "Why Aren't There More Women Leaders in Academic

Medicine? The Views of Clinical Department Chairs," *Academic Medicine* 76, no. 5 (2001): 453–465.

4. Ash et al., "Compensation and Advancement"; and C. Laine and B.J. Turner, "Unequal Pay for Equal Work: The Gender Gap in Academic Medicine," *Annals of Internal Medicine* 141, no. 3 (2004): 238–240.

5. W. Levinson, K. Kaufman, and J. Bickel, "Part-Time Faculty in Academic Medicine: Present Status and Future Challenges," *Annals of Internal Medicine* 119, no. 3 (1993): 220–225; and P.L. Carr, K.C. Gareis, and R.C. Barnett, "Characteristics and Outcomes for Women Physicians Who Work Reduced Hours," *Journal of Women's Health* 12, no. 4 (2003): 399–405.

6. R. Wilson and P. Fogg, "On Parental Leave, Men Have It Easier," *Chronicle of Higher Education* 51, no. 18 (2005): 25.

7. P.L. Carr et al. "Relation of Family Responsibilities and Gender to the Productivity and Career Satisfaction of Medical Faculty," *Annals of Internal Medicine* 129, no. 7 (1998): 532–538.

8. Yedidia and Bickel, "Why Aren't There More Women Leaders in Academic Medicine?"

9. S.J. Correll, S. Benard, and I. Paik, "Getting a Job: Is There a Mother-hood Penalty?" *American Journal of Sociology* 112, no. 5 (2007): 1297–1338.

10. E. Wulfhorst, "Study: U.S. Mothers Deserve $134,121 in Salary," *Boston Globe*, 5 May 2006.

11. U.S. Department of Labor, Bureau of Labor Statistics, "American Time Use Survey Summary," 28 June 2007, http://www.bls.gov/news.release/atus.nr0.htm (accessed 12 December 2007).

12. L. Belkin, "The Opt-Out Revolution," *New York Times*, 26 October 2003.

13. J.C. Williams, "'Opt Out' or Pushed Out? How the Press Covers Work/Family Conflict: The Untold Story of Why Women Leave the Workforce" (San Francisco: University of California, Hastings College of the Law, October 2006).

14. B.A. McBride, S.J. Schoppe-Sullivan, and M. Ho, "The Mediating Role of Fathers' School Involvement on Student Achievement," *Journal of Applied Developmental Psychology* 26, no. 2 (2005): 201–216; and J.T. Downer and J.L. Mendez, "African American Father Involvement and Preschool Children's Social Readiness," *Early Education and Development* 16, no. 3 (2005): 317–340.

Disorientation

By Alok A. Khorana

From *Health Affairs*

THERE IS SNOW outside the kitchen door. It covers the deck in white sheets, unbroken except for the occasional paw print, and it cascades off the steps in thick, soft layers onto the pine trees in our backyard. Inside, our home hums with the usual Sunday evening flurry of activity. My wife is coordinating dinner with homework—both hers and the children's. In the background, I hear my two-year-old son trying to entice the dog to sit by offering her a treat. This is no small task, given that the dog weighs nearly three times as much as he does. But he has learnt early to stand ground before his three older siblings—my stepsons—who both tower over him and dote on him, and he is practicing this skill on the dog with some flair.

I contemplate the busy week ahead: a looming grant submission deadline, a talk to second-year medical students, a day trip to a nearby cancer center to give a research talk. And, of course, patients. I help run a busy gastrointestinal oncology program (a subspecialty within a subspecialty), and my overflowing clinics threaten to spill onto all other parts of my job.

All of this—a life of academia, of family, of life in snowy upstate New York—is in one sense routine, ordinary even. But when my mind takes pause, it is always with a sense of wonderment at what distances have been traveled, what has been achieved, and what has been left behind.

Here and There

I arrived in upstate New York in the summer of 1996, just a few months past my twenty-fourth birthday. I was eighteen days late for the start of my residency in internal medicine, and, as a consequence, I had missed intern orientation day. Whoever set the schedule didn't seem to view this as being particularly a problem, as my very first weekend in town I was assigned to be the night float intern.

I spent the day preparing for my first night of working in an American hospital. I acquired a stethoscope, scrubs, and a lab coat and went over the resuscitation protocols. Summer in Buffalo—unlike summer in India—is a beautiful season. The trees are full of luscious green leaves, there are flowers in every dooryard, the sun doesn't set until late evening, and there is a certain liveliness to the city—as if it is trying to make up for all those lost winter months. I remember finding this cheery atmosphere somewhat incongruent with the dread that I felt as I walked the short distance across the street from the studio apartment I had just rented and into the stone and glass entrance of Millard Fillmore Hospital.

Entering it that night, I was no different—at least on paper—from the thousands of other interns who had started at hundreds of hospitals throughout the country that June of

1996. I had finished medical school; I had studied for and passed the United States Medical Licensing Exam Steps 1 and 2; I had been interviewed in person earlier that year at multiple residency programs; and, after a rigorous matching process, I had been selected as one of the twelve interns starting that year in the Buffalo program. The only items that set me apart were that I was not a U.S. citizen and that I had graduated from a foreign medical school.

That was on paper.

In terms of practical experience, however, it was an entirely different matter. I had, indeed, completed medical school and even started an internship in internal medicine. But I had done so in a setting so removed from the gleaming U.S. hospital that I was walking into as to belong to a different world. At the time, most students and residents in India received their training primarily in understaffed, inadequately funded public hospitals that provided free care to mostly poor patients. The ward of the public hospital that I worked in until just a few months before was located in a dilapidated two-story building. Its windows were festooned with colorful saris hung out to dry by patients and their relatives. Inside, thirty to forty patients were housed in two large rooms, their beds separated only by a distance of a few feet. The only concession to privacy was separate large rooms for male and female patients. Every week my resident/attending physician team was responsible for one twenty-four-hour period (an "admit day") when all sick patients seen either in clinic or in the emergency room would be admitted under our care. On a busy admit day, even the space between beds would fill up with floor mattresses housing "overflow" patients.

As a first-year resident, I was the person on first call for these patients all day, every night, all 365 days of the year. (The U.S. term "night float" was—for lack of a better term—a foreign concept.) I had exactly two nurses to help me. I would typically spend all day in the ward as outpatients were sent in by my senior residents and attending physician. My day would be occupied

writing notes, ordering tests, and performing a variety of procedures, including taps to remove fluid around the chest wall
and abdomen, even liver biopsies. On occasion, I would also
have to help the nurses with difficult intravenous line or urinary
catheter placements. At night, I also doubled as a laboratory
assistant, counting leukocytes and looking for malarial parasites
in peripheral smears. Early in the morning, having had little
to no sleep, I would do rounds on each patient with my senior
resident. These rounds, in keeping with the hierarchical Indian
system, could best be described as confrontational: I would be
challenged on every diagnosis or decision I had made through
the night. An hour later, this would be repeated, but with my
resident presenting and defending our decisions and our attending physician the one doing the challenging.

In many ways, therefore, I was better prepared than most
U.S. medical students starting a residency program. I was used to
being independent, I had already performed more procedures
than most trainees would conduct through the course of their
entire residency, I had confidence in my physical examination
skills because we'd had to "make do" without access to expensive
diagnostic tests, and I had learnt to think quickly on my feet.

But I had never worked a single day in a U.S. hospital.

I had never used a pager or answered a page, never looked
up labs on a computer screen, never dictated a note, never been
exposed to American patients' expectations of privacy and medical information, never dealt with discharge planning or nursing
home placement or insurance issues.

The First Night On Call

So it was with trepidation that I walked that night into the physicians lounge in Buffalo and paged the on-call intern to let him
know that I was here. Ian showed up a few minutes later looking
a little harassed. "It's been a busy afternoon," he said, "Here's
the sign-out."

I didn't know what a sign-out was, but it appeared from the crumpled sheet in his hand that it was a list of patients who I would be responsible for through the night. "Cool," I said, acting as if I had done this a hundred times before.

Ian went quickly through the list of patients, and it was pretty apparent that these were not the diagnoses I was used to dealing with; the list included patients with emphysema, acute bronchitis, stroke, and even a few chronic ventilator-dependent patients. I confessed to Ian that it was my first night working here, although I didn't tell him how different the hospital and its patients were from anything I had ever experienced before.

"Well," he said, with only a hurried note of sympathy in his voice, "ask the nurses for advice—they've been doing this way longer than you or I have. Make sure you use your intern survival guide and pocket drug manual. Good luck."

And he was gone before I could summon the courage to tell him that, having missed orientation day, I possessed neither handbook.

I used Ian's advice on the first page I received, a call about ventilator settings on a chronic ventilator-dependent patient.

"What do you suggest?" I asked the nurse who had called me, and then agreed with her recommendations. There were a couple more pages that I also dispensed with relatively success-fully, and I felt myself grow a little confident in my answers.

Then I got called to the floor to see my first patient. She was in her seventies, had recently undergone surgery, and was complaining of pain at the operation site. The discussion that ensued with the nurse was the low point of my night, and pos-sibly of my entire intern year.

"She needs something for pain," said the nurse.

"How about ibuprofen?" I suggested, trying out an authori-tative tone.

"She's allergic to ibuprofen," replied the nurse, patiently. "Says so right in front of the chart."

At this point, I decided to forgo my newly acquired authoritativeness and fell back on Ian's advice.

"What do *you* suggest?"

"How about Tylenol?"

Tylenol. Tylenol. It was something in the way she said it, how easily the word slipped off her tongue, or perhaps the tone of her voice, that implied an obviousness to the suggestion. Trouble was, although the term seemed vaguely familiar, *for the life of me I couldn't remember what Tylenol was*. In my defense, I should point out that the popular brand name for acetaminophen in India is Crocin, and Tylenol had never been marketed there. I had seen commercials on American television for Tylenol when I did my residency interviews a few months earlier, but I hadn't paid close enough attention to see what generic drug was being advertised. I hadn't bought any in the short time I had been in the U.S. because, like any good immigrant physician, I arrived with my suitcase packed with a variety of drug samples designed to meet any foreseeable calamity.

I fought the voices in my head that were screaming at me to drop the ruse, quit pretending that I could do this—be an American doctor—and board the first flight back home. And I came up with a gem of an excuse.

"I don't have my pocket drug manual; I'm not sure what the dose is."

"Its 650 milligrams PO q 4–6 hrs PRN, *doctor*," she replied. She said it with a twinkle in her eye, though.

Which wasn't much reassurance a few minutes later when I located a drug compendium and discovered exactly how much of a faux pas it was to ask about "dosing" a Tylenol tablet.

Transition

I made it through that night, and none of my patients died or went to the intensive care unit, which is the definition of a successful intern, as Ian pointed out to me the next morning. The nurse who had provided me with the Tylenol recommendation was discreet; no rumors about the doctor who didn't know how to dose Tylenol followed me on my next rotation. (She would, periodically, tease me about it—and she brought it up again on my last day as a resident three years later. So clearly that night left quite an impression on her. I never did confess to her—or to anyone but my wife before now—that it wasn't just the dose of Tylenol that I was unaware of.)

It is important to note that I was hardly alone in undergoing this transition to becoming an American physician. Indeed, arriving in the mid-1990s, I was part of a massive wave of immigrant physician trainees, many of whom stayed on and are practicing in the United States. In 2006 nearly a quarter-million U.S. physicians were international medical graduates, or IMGs, accounting for 25.3 percent of the total physician count. By one estimate, as many as 44 percent of all foreign health care workers arrived in the U.S. after 1990, as did I. Also, I was fairly representative: I had graduated from a medical school in India (Indian physicians account for one-fifth of all IMGs), specialized in internal medicine (one-third of all internists are IMGs), and settled in New York State (42 percent of physicians in New York are IMGs).

Yet despite these large numbers, most residency programs do not have formal orientation or acculturation programs in place for IMG residents (nor did they then). In part, this might be because programs wish to avoid the appearance of discrimination, and selecting out IMG residents for special training is at odds with this goal. But so much of medicine relies on verbal and non-verbal communication. It is not difficult to imagine minor miscommunications leading to errors: some simple, others causing physician mistrust, and even some with major health consequences. Only recently, the Educational Commission for Foreign Medical Graduates (ECFMG) and some residency programs—often at the urging of IMGs who later joined as faculty or IMG leaders within the American College of Physicians—have begun to institute orientation programs specifically for IMGs starting internships. This standard needs to be widely adopted across all residency programs, perhaps with a national mandate from the Accreditation Council for Graduate Medical Education (ACGME) working jointly with the ECFMG.

Life got easier over the successive weeks and months. I discovered that American patients expected competence and compassion from their physicians. And, in this, they were no different than the patients in India that I had taken care of. Life also got easier on a personal level: I found friends among the other interns, nurses, and attending physicians on the hospital staff—both American and immigrant. It really gives you a sense of our shared humanity—how much we are like each other— when an Indian intern, a Jordanian intern, and an American intern can meet for coffee after rounds and have the exact same gripe about their resident.

I have now completed more than a decade in the United States since that first night as an intern. This past decade has been marked by the usual upheavals of life magnified by my decision to call two places, separated by half a globe, home. The successive deaths of my parents and my inability to be there for them have been especially hard. But there have been rewards. In particular, my American wife and the blended American family that we raise together have allowed me to be open to the world and to others in ways that were previously closed to my insular way of thinking. My patients, too, have made me feel part of a family, trusting me with intimate details of their lives, sharing in my own highs and lows, writing notes and calling when I lost my father, bringing gifts for our newborn.

Have there been less welcoming aspects to my immigrant story? Yes, of course; some felt more keenly than others. Such as when I discovered that institutional regulatory authorities record the percentage of IMGs in training programs as an adverse quality indicator. Or the time when I was passed over by a certain prestigious medical center for fellowship training, yet a less qualified European IMG physician was welcomed. Even amongst IMGs, there are degrees to foreignness, as physician-author Abraham Verghese has pointed out. But episodes like this have been, for the most part, minor irritants. When I have been assessed by the faculty at my residency and fellowship programs, when I have been offered faculty positions or promotions, when my grant applications have been evaluated on their scientific merits and demerits, I have never felt unfairly judged.

We don't say this often enough as immigrants.

We don't say it primarily because if you're trying to assimilate, it is almost a requirement that you adopt the cynical, ironic American conversational tone. But the truth of the matter is that—unlike most other nations—America always has been and, almost as important, perceives itself to be, an immigrant nation. What this means is that, for us immigrants, the United States is a generous and welcoming country, and Americans are, for the most part, a generous and welcoming and forgiving people.

Forgiving, even of a doctor who doesn't know what Tylenol is.

Lessons from an Emergency Room Nightmare

Harold Pollack

from the *American Prospect*

I HELD MY wife Veronica's hand as the technician applied cool gel to her chest. At first, the ultrasound images were the fuzzy black-and-whites I remembered from before our daughters Rebecca and Hannah were born. After a few touches to the LCD screen, a breathtaking three-dimensional movie began to run. It featured Veronica's heart, its thick walls beating yellow against a black background.

The technician maneuvered a trackball to reveal the various parts undulating in unison. Colored regions displayed blood velocity and turbulence through the different chambers. Suspended in virtual space, Veronica's heart looked every millimeter the impregnable pump I had always assumed it was.

Veronica is 46, does four hard workouts every week on the stepping machine, eats sensibly, and has a resting pulse of 60. So when she woke me at 2 A.M. and calmly reported funny chest pains radiating to her shoulder blades and down her arms, the obvious came to mind, but it was hard to really believe. Veronica and Rebecca had been coughing and feverish for a week. The three of us had embarrassing cold sores. Acid reflux, a sore diaphragm—anything seemed more likely than a heart attack.

You need a hard head and a soft heart to manage a loved one's medical emergency. It's surprisingly easy for smart people to be nudged by circumstance and human frailty into doing careless or foolish things. We had two sleeping daughters across the hall. The thought of them waking up to flashing ambulance lights was daunting. We worried about leaving them or dragging them to an emergency room. Still, Veronica had never felt anything like this. We had to do something. So we threw on some clothes, and drove to the 24-hour urgent-care center a half-mile from our house.

SEVERAL PEOPLE MADE mistakes in Veronica's care. The worst and most deadly mistake was ours: going to this urgent-care center. Veronica's symptoms demanded a 911 call. I knew better—or I certainly should have. I am a certified expert, director of the University of Chicago Center for Health Administration Studies. I've served on expert panels of the Institute of Medicine, no less.

I was swayed to discount what was happening—Veronica, a clinical nurse specialist, was, too—by disbelief, by her recent illness, and by her general fitness. We were also swayed by the expected hassle and expense of an ER visit. We envisioned paying a large bill to be prescribed some Tums. Last year, Veronica went out-of-network for urgent care. That cost $700.

In part, we hesitated because that was exactly what the modern health-insurance system is designed to make us do. A quarter-century ago, the RAND Health Insurance Experiment

(HIE) established the basic argument for deductibles and co-payments in insurance. HIE remains the most important policy experiment in American history. Its most potent finding was that people who got free care used 40 percent more services than did others assigned to cost-sharing plans. Yet the free care produced little measurable additional benefit for the average patient. These results are often cited in support of co-payments and deductibles designed to discourage inappropriate care. Policy-makers and payers are particularly concerned about the real and alleged over-use of emergency care. Charging higher co-payments is one obvious response.

It seems counterintuitive that demand for ER services would be sensitive to price. If you slice off your finger with a steak knife, you won't be thinking about the money. Yet it turns out that many ailments—Veronica's included—are ambiguous, and so price matters. RAND investigators found that individuals in cost-sharing plans reduced ER use by one-third when compared with the free-care group.

Co-payments did discourage wasteful use among HIE participants. ER visits in relatively non-urgent categories such as sprains and back pain were 47 percent less frequent in cost-sharing plans. Unfortunately, co-payments also discouraged appropriate use. Participants enrolled in the cost-sharing plans were 23 percent less likely to seek ER care for "more urgent" problems, including fractures and asthma.

Most patients cannot reliably distinguish appropriate from inappropriate ER use. In many cases, even experts find the distinction fuzzy. I once co-wrote a study of a managed behavioral health plan that imposed a 50 percent co-payment on psychiatric ER visits. Do we really want to impose these barriers? When someone feels that funny chest pain, how long do we want her to dither before seeking help?

Veronica and I made a critical decision in choosing the urgent-care clinic. Your first medical provider in an emergency determines who will frame the initial hypotheses of your illness, who will coordinate your care, and, often, the person who hears the cleanest direct account of what is wrong. I had never been inside this imposing structure, which advertises and charges as an emergency-department affiliate of a local hospital. We arrived to find it nearly empty. The staff promptly took an electrocardiogram (EKG) that looked normal and administered aspirin and nitroglycerin. Veronica took a gastrointestinal cocktail of antacid and lidocaine in case this was acid reflux. It seemed to help, which I found reassuring. They administered a chest X-ray. After bumpy preliminaries, they administered the standard cardiac-enzyme tests.

Key enzyme levels were very high, indicating that heart cells had died and had released their hidden proteins. Yet the staff remained unsure that the test equipment was working. As the tests were rerun, the staff tried to administer a CT scan, but the intravenous dye infiltrated into Veronica's forearm, causing excruciating pain.

I remained convinced this was all an annoying set of benign, if painful, screw-ups.

I CANNOT SAY why I was not more forceful in getting Veronica out of there. Throughout, she seemed fine, talking normally, except that her chest, and then her arm, really hurt. My alarm steadily increased as the realization sank in that something could be genuinely amiss. An amazing four hours after arriving, we received the repeated enzyme tests. That's when the ambulance was called to transport Veronica to a real hospital. I gingerly asked the doctor about taking her to the big university hospital one hour away. He replied, quite reasonably, that there was no time. I raced home and drove the kids to a friend's house.

At the hospital, an emergency-room doctor stated without preliminaries: "Bottom line—you've had a heart attack." The enzyme tests were definitive. Fortunately there was no other detectable damage. He explained that this was the kind of heart attack, more common than one would suppose, that can leave no obvious damage. A tiny piece of plaque becomes dislodged, initiating clotting. Such an attack can be essentially self-healing once it runs its course. I gave the gruff but comfortably authoritative cardiologist the business card of Veronica's internist and asked him to call.

Veronica needed cardiac catheterization. This is a delicate procedure. Cardiologists and their surgical teams differ substantially in skill and in post-operative mortality. For 25 years, health-services researchers have documented that it's good to have an operation in the right hospital by the right people. Many jurisdictions have begun to publish hospital-specific and surgeon-specific rankings of observed and expected mortality rates for these procedures.

As you might imagine, ranking is a complicated subject. Hospitals complain they are penalized because they serve high-risk, complex patients. Hospitals may also game things. There is suggestive evidence that cardiac report cards encourage physicians to provide less-aggressive treatment to minority patients and others who tend to have worse outcomes. Risk-adjustment methods developed to address these concerns have spurred needed changes. A striking number of surgeons in the highest mortality categories retired or moved away when New York implemented report-card systems. A 2006 Health Affairs paper by Ashish Jha and Arnold Epstein reports: "With the release of each report card, approximately one in five bottom-quartile surgeons relocated or ceased practicing within two years." New York's post-operative mortality rates sharply declined after ratings were published. Rankings were not the only reasons for improvement, but they helped.

Not surprisingly, high-volume facilities perform better. Surgeons get better with practice. Care teams get better at minimizing post-operative infections. Some hospitals become popular because they are good; others become good because they are popular. Which came first? If you're a patient, you don't care. There are ongoing debates over whether cardiac catheterization and other delicate services should be provided by a small number of high-volume regional centers. Probably they should, though this is hard to pull off in our decentralized and competitive system. The data also reveal surprising disparities, sometimes between adjoining hospitals or those we might otherwise consider peers.

New York state publishes risk-adjusted 30-day mortality rankings. Based on 2003–2005 data (released last February), where would you want your ambulance to go in the New York area? You might not guess that Bellevue Hospital and the Long Island Jewish Hospital performed markedly better than many more famous hospitals. You might not suspect that Montefiore-Einstein Heart Center ranked poorly in both mortality and post-operative complication.

I have presented this information to hundreds of students at Yale, the University of Michigan, and the University of Chicago. I could cite a wealth of data on many topics. Yet when Veronica got sick, my personal databank included nothing on the hospitals near my own home. You don't comparison shop alongside a loved one's hospital gurney.

As the bedside conversation proceeded, I wondered whether to sell our house. I wasn't thinking about the sub-prime mess. I just wanted to live near a great cardiac facility. A classic analysis by Mark McLellan, Barbara McNeil, and Joseph Newhouse showed that people who happen to live near these hospitals were more likely to survive cardiac emergencies. I wish I had taken that paper to heart.

The community hospital that treated Veronica is, by reputation, probably the best within 10 miles of us. The attending cardiologist is well respected and projected an infectious certainty about what was wrong, how to fix it, and who was in charge. I found his decisiveness reassuring. Still, I would rather have had this performed at a major academic medical center or at least done by someone I had vetted. I again rather awkwardly asked the emergency-room docs whether Veronica should be moved.

I called a friend who is a good internist who said they seemed to be doing sensible things, and there was no time to screw around moving her. Given the situation, there was nothing else to do.

The team whisked Veronica upstairs for the angiogram. They threaded a catheter into her groin area and ran it up near the heart to examine arteries that might have been blocked. I sat pensively in the waiting area. The cardiologist shortly emerged to report that the angiogram had gone well. There was no observable tissue damage. There were no blockages. Her arteries were squeaky clean.

Days later, I looked up the local rankings. Our hospital wasn't ranked badly. Its cardiac catheterization is 40 percent cheaper than the fancy university hospital I preferred. The bad news: Its post-operative mortality rate was 40 percent higher than that of another community hospital I never held in much regard three miles from our home.

THE VARIOUS WAITING rooms were especially sobering. Dozens of tight-lipped people filled them, worried, first and foremost, about their loved ones. The hospital is located in a gritty South Chicago suburb. Many of the people sitting with me were surely wondering, how will I pay for this?

I wasn't worrying about money. I remember thinking: Thank God we have good insurance. At least I think we do. Six months later, I still don't know how much this episode will ultimately cost. I am confident we will not go medically bankrupt, as many patients do with limited or no insurance. Jonathan Cohn's book Sick describes Chicagoans' struggles with medical debt, including a poor, semi-retired nun sued by a Catholic health system. Sitting in that waiting room, I was also struck by the responsibility each of us has to care for our mind and body. We are vulnerable to genetics and bad luck. Still, the intensive care unit brutally displays the consequences of poor health behaviors. Surprising numbers of young people are there, suffering and sometimes dying when this doesn't have to be.

It was hard not to notice something else. That waiting room, like so many others I have frequented in my 15 years in public health, was filled with people of color. Public perceptions of racial and ethnic disparities are shaped by headlines about homicide, substance abuse, infant mortality, AIDS. Mundane cardiovascular diseases exact a far heavier toll in minority communities, within which child and adult obesity have markedly worsened. I fear that waiting rooms may need more chairs.

Within a few hours after the angiogram, Veronica was in intensive care, and we began to digest the bizarre news. Once the anesthesia wore off, she felt real chest pain but was otherwise amazingly normal. Wired up to the monitors, she was soon sitting up doing her cross-stitch, joking with my sister, asking about the kids. An infectious-disease specialist came through and treated her cold sores. Things became boring.

Veronica stayed in that ICU for three days. A pneumatic messaging tube thwonked loudly and randomly throughout the night. Various machines would beep if Veronica moved her arm and impinged on some tubing. On top of that, Veronica was in pain, which the cardiologist explained later was a normal reaction to blood returning to the damaged heart areas. The effect is grueling. Sleep disruption is a prominent cause of what is charmingly labeled "ICU psychosis." Despite that, the staff provided much wonderful care. A community-hospital ICU resembles what hospital care often used to be: kind nurses in an unhurried environment where they could pay close attention to patients.

Veronica spent her last 24 hours in that hospital on a regular floor. Fewer nurses were responsible for more sick patients. Veronica was in pretty good shape by then. She saw her nurse one or two times, not much more. The cardiologist and the local attending shook our hands, assured Veronica she would be fine, and sent us packing.

I was nervous but happy to bring Veronica home. Forty-eight hours earlier, she had been wired up in a cardiac ICU; now no medical provider seemed all that interested in seeing her. We made an appointment to see the cardiologist nearly one month later. We called Veronica's young university internist. I would have thought the words: "I had a heart attack" would provide some scheduling advantage—apparently not. The medical center is de-emphasizing primary care. It's hard to make money on these services in a tertiary-care setting. During the 10 days before we saw the internist, Veronica dutifully took her medications and set about recovering from her illness and from the grueling days in the hospital. Recovery was slow. She had trouble climbing stairs, got winded a lot, and needed a lot of sleep.

Internists have taken some hits in recent years. A New York Times story in March noted that dermatologists earn twice as much and work 10 fewer hours per week. The Times quotes an aspiring dermatologist as saying that internal medicine is "viewed as easy because anyone can get into it." Since preventive medical care cases can be "humdrum," he said there is a "lack of respect for what they do."

ALTHOUGH THAT STUDENT doesn't know it, internists are the linchpin of our medical system. As described in Jerome Groopman's beautiful book How Doctors Think, physicians make sense of a disorganized jumble of data, recognize latent signs of trouble, chase down patterns when things don't look right, and help patients form a coordinated care plan. Veronica's internist started the 30-minute appointment with a jaw-dropper: "I want to hear what happened straight from you. I should say at the outset that I don't think you've had a heart attack."

Before the appointment, he had mastered Veronica's hospital record. That already put him miles ahead of most other doctors. It just didn't look right that a healthy gym rat would have a sudden heart attack with no warning and no detectable damage. He had a hunch, which he checked out with five or six senior colleagues. They agreed that a viral infection of the heart, viral myocarditis, was more likely.

He took an EKG, which revealed Veronica's resting pulse of 47. She had previously been so fit that her normal heart rate was already quite low. The beta-blocker Veronica had been prescribed was too potent, and nobody was monitoring it—making her one of many people who become sick from their medication. Mercifully, the internist tapered the beta-blocker. He also arranged for an echocardiogram in order to make a more definitive diagnosis. That echocardiogram is where this article began.

Two days after the echo, we sat in an examining room with a university cardiologist, a wonderfully effervescent, small man with a flowing gray beard and an Irish brogue. My heart initially sank when he said, "I have not read your chart. I want to hear from you." He proceeded to ask Veronica in detail about everything that had happened. Veronica tried to be efficient and precise to fit the confines of our visit. "Slow down," he said. "We have plenty of time. Did the cardiologist say your arteries look 'clean,' or 'squeaky clean'?"

After 15 or 30 minutes of questions, he said, "OK. I am going to stop the conversation now, and I am going to read your records." He methodically reviewed what had been written. "Your internist has written a Bible about you," he happily noted. He went through all the lab values and commented almost flirtatiously: "You have the kidneys of a young girl."

After more back-and-forth, he noted the competing hypotheses. He then looked over the echocardiogram results and said, "This is a classic presentation of viral myocarditis." He noted that a damaging heart attack would have shown a dead or damaged region, too weakened to support the heart's syncopated beat. I cannot imagine what cardiac patients experience when they watch live movies of their own hearts in visibly damaged condition.

My own heart skipped when he said to Veronica: "Your echo clearly shows a heart pumping poorly from the myocarditis." It wasn't just the beta-blockers that were making her winded. Her right atrium was enlarged.

As this article goes to print, Veronica is doing well but is facing a nine-month recovery. We have one loose end. Veronica's university-hospital record says that she is on aspirin and a blood thinner and that she is recovering from viral myocarditis. Yet if she falls ill tonight, an ambulance will deliver her to that community hospital, whose records indicate that she is a recovering heart-attack patient taking a potent dose of beta-blockers. Nothing in our health-care system reliably reconciles these different versions of reality. Everyone involved seems skittish to close this loop. What will we tell her original cardiologist? Will he worry that we will sue? Will he argue with us or with the other guy?

PEOPLE DRAW THEIR own lessons from intense experiences. Perhaps most frightening is the ease with which smart people make bad mistakes and never look back. Cognitive psychologists have documented the impact of imperfect heuristics and biases on medical decisions. It is hard to overstate the power of getting stuck in a groove, particularly when psychological crosswinds or workplace pressures distort our thinking. A wealth of data confirms this observation when we are driving a car, buying a home, or diagnosing a seriously ill patient. Such findings provide a human frame through which to view many mistakes in Veronica's care, including mine.

Our community hospital did a great job that first day. The cardiologist performed an expert angiogram. We are grateful, even knowing that they overlooked the myocarditis when Veronica's presentation cried out for this diagnosis. She had recently experienced a bad viral infection. She had no sign of artery or heart tissue damage consistent with a heart attack. Every doctor I know has said: Yup, of course, viral infection.

Medical errors seem more egregious in hindsight than they actually are. Groopman's How Doctors Think recounts many serious mistakes but also several heroic diagnoses made when doctors spot things others have missed. But many of these cases just don't seem that hard: the chronic anorexia that turns out to be celiac disease, the ER patient with chest pain who turns out to have unstable angina, the overlooked infected abscess. These examples are frightening because they reveal how skilled professionals go astray.

I can't say why Veronica's doctors missed her heart infection, but I have some clues. For one thing, Veronica's doctors never performed an echocardiogram. Such missed opportunities are common. Tejal Gandhi of Brigham and Women's Hospital and colleagues recently examined closed malpractice cases involving missed or delayed diagnoses. More than half included some failure to order an appropriate diagnostic test. This pattern may be hard to generalize. Only a tiny proportion of medical mistakes and injuries result in malpractice claims. Moreover, a missed diagnostic test is an especially provable form of malpractice.

Emergency physicians face disconcerting challenges that make them especially vulnerable to cognitive error. They must act decisively based on what is currently suspected or known. Doctors and patients both want certainty in an anxious situation. No one is reassured when the doctor says, "I'm not sure what's wrong." Yet those same doctors must remember that their provisional hypotheses might be wrong.

That openness is hard to sustain over the hours and days in which everyone's thinking becomes anchored in a specific diagnosis. The possibility of heart attack was on everyone's mind based on Veronica's dramatic cardiac-enzyme numbers. Had we gone to the hospital first rather than to the urgent-care center, the staff might have conducted a more reflective conversation with Veronica about the specific history of her illness. Given her urgent-care admission, Veronica needed an immediate angiogram before that conversation could really be had. In those first few hours, heart attack was the most reasonable working hypothesis. This deadly possibility needed immediate attention. Yet as economists and psychologists could readily predict, confirmation bias distorted subsequent judgments.

Later, things became murkier. Veronica's arteries and heart tissue looked fine. Her only symptoms were the bad enzyme results and continued chest and arm pain. These were consistent with a heart attack but also with other things. Healthy, 46-year-old women rarely have heart attacks that refuse to leave a trace. That pattern would later pique the curiosity of Veronica's internist. In the moment, hospital staff seemed stuck in a groove created by their own initial treatment plan. Their real mistake was to be incurious once the immediate crisis had passed.

Here's where the need for systemic thinking becomes apparent. When a tired doctor writes an extra zero on his prescription pad or makes a bad initial call, the result can be catastrophic, but it doesn't have to be. Hospitals can be organized to acknowledge the reality that doctors make mistakes and have messy handwriting, and that busy nurses make mistakes, too. As Jerome Groopman knows as a doctor, these mistakes are part of the landscape of medical care.

But Groopman's perspective shows its limitations. He focuses on how clinicians can avoid predictable errors and cognitive distortions. Yet as pediatric cardiologist Darshak Sanghavi notes, diagnostic errors reflect faulty systems as much as they reflect faulty thinking by any one specific person. When we consider how a decent community hospital can improve care, it may be most useful to ask not how doctors think but how systems think.

Writing in the *New Yorker*, another physician/journalist, Atul Gawande, has noted the value of simple checklists in matters such as controlling hospital infection. Standardization helps individual clinicians to avoid errors. It also forces hospitals and health-care systems to scrutinize their procedures and habits when elements of that checklist are frequently left undone. It's not glamorous, but this is how large organizations improve their performance. One can also create practices and protocols that reduce the likelihood and the probable consequences of common diagnostic errors. Suppose a hospital established a simple rule: Every cardiac patient who reports a recent infection should receive an echocardiogram. Such a rule or a more refined alternative would probably have saved us much time and trouble.

Some things can't be easily replicated. Our internist brought a fresh perspective, distanced from the initial emergency. Equally important, he operated in a hallway culture that encourages questioning and provides backup when things don't add up. He could ask several smart colleagues about what might have been missed. That's a key advantage of academic medicine.

Given my health-policy credentials, I'm embarrassed that I navigated this emergency relatively badly and generally felt no less bewildered than anyone else. I guess the final lessons are more personal. We must forgive ourselves, and others, for our near-misses. Then we must learn from these experiences.

America's AIDS Apartheid

Kai Wright

From *American Prospect*

The domestic HIV/AIDS epidemic is increasingly black and Southern—and spiraling out of control.

THE HOPE IN Tracy's voice was contagious. He had just come out of Alabama's state prison system and was looking forward to starting over. He'd gotten some part-time work and secured a comfortable, if sparsely furnished apartment. He was a classic Southern hunk—a handsome, stout, mocha-skinned man with a slow drawl and a natural charm—and so had no trouble finding women to date. That was exciting but also scary, because Tracy had newly committed himself to confronting his 12-year-old HIV infection.

He beamed with pride at the progress he was making. "I talked to one," he bashfully boasted to me about his coming-out process to would-be girlfriends. She'd been pressuring him to have sex, and he knew he had to disclose first. "She appreciated my honesty." Things were going well.

I wanted to be hopeful for Tracy, too. After more than a decade of writing about AIDS, I've come to recognize the liberated look on his face—the relief that shines in someone's eyes when he gives up on fear and shame and starts figuring out how to live with—rather than in spite of—an HIV diagnosis. But I knew Tracy would get little help on what was going to be a hard road to wellness, because his story arc is sadly typical of the epidemic that is now raging around him—years of denial masquerading as optimism, followed by a mad scramble to patch things up when it's already too late.

Tracy was diagnosed back in 1993, the first time he went into lockup. He got no counseling and no treatment, just the news that he was HIV–positive. He was outwardly healthy so, not surprisingly, he ignored this piece of overwhelming, incomprehensible information and went on with his life, bouncing in and out of jail. It wasn't until 2005, the year I met him, that Tracy finally came to understand the gravity of his situation. He'd gotten some education during his last stint in prison, after activists sued the state and forced it to provide meaningful care to the HIV–positive inmates. Who knows how many others he passed on the virus to in the interim. But to focus on missed HIV–prevention opportunities is crazy-making; they are too many to count. What mattered as I listened to Tracy describe his future was that, finally, he preferred reality to the false comfort of denial. That's more than I can say for both the federal and state-level response to the fast-growing ranks of people like him.

America declared a terribly premature victory over AIDS more than a decade ago, when new treatment regimens hit the market and dramatically halted the parade of young funerals. And there's no denying the progress: Today's death rate is a small fraction of what it was then. But controlling an epidemic isn't the same as ending it. We confused the two achievements and turned our attention to epidemics overseas. We've spent years watching with sympathetic awe as infection rates have spiraled upward in places like sub-Saharan Africa, where people have struggled to afford the lifesaving drugs we assume are readily available here at home. All the while, the U.S. epidemic has been barreling toward the precipice.

More Americans are living with HIV today than ever before—an estimated 1.2 million—and the number is increasing by tens of thousands annually. Worse, there's every reason to believe the problem is exponentially graver than we know. AIDS researchers and service providers have been anxiously awaiting a U.S. Centers for Disease Control and Prevention (CDC) study that is expected to find the epidemic to be far larger than believed. Yet, over the last eight years policy-makers have so neglected the care system that we cobbled together in the 1990s to control the epidemic that people have died, right here in America, while lingering on treatment waiting lists like those in the developing world.

Meanwhile, an AIDS apartheid has hardened here. John Edwards' two Americas are perhaps most clearly witnessed in the waiting rooms of AIDS clinics around the country. African Americans, who are 13 percent of the U.S. population, now account for a stunning half of all people living with HIV/AIDS and half of all those newly infected every year. The numbers are even more shocking when you look at the people among whom the virus is spreading most quickly. One depressing study of gay and bisexual men in five large U.S. cities found 46 percent of black men to already be positive. *Nearly half.* No population on Earth has registered infection rates that high.

Nowhere is this crisis more acute than in the southeast United States. What was once considered an urban, coastal epidemic—centered in gay havens like New York City, San Francisco, and Los Angeles—is now a surprisingly rural, Southern one. More than half of all new infections logged between 2001 and 2004 were found in the South. Those infections are far more likely to be found among Southerners who are black, low-income, and diagnosed with advanced conditions they do not have the resources to control.

Yet Southern state governments have only recently begun to understand that they preside over the new ground zero for America's AIDS epidemic. The AIDS clinic Tracy turned to for care was the only one serving the entire southeastern quadrant of Alabama. The clinic's efforts are heroic, but the thin network it has built is hardly enough to absorb demand in an area that's home to the state's highest per capita HIV–infection rate. That's sadly typical of the region. If the AIDS–care safety net is in tatters nationally, in many Southern states it never existed in the first place. Nearly three decades after the epidemic's start, America has so squandered its successes that we will have to entirely re-create them—or face a return to the days of the costly, painful, and needless deaths of thousands.

AIDS HAS HAD a racially lopsided impact on America from the start. African Americans accounted for roughly a quarter of AIDS deaths as early as 1985. But the definitive cleaving of AIDS into two epidemics came about a decade later, when a remarkable scientific breakthrough turned HIV infection into a manageable, if lifelong condition—for those with access to treatment.

The first AIDS drug, known as AZT, didn't hit the market until the latter half of the 1980s. AZT was actually first developed in 1964, through cancer research funded by the National Institutes of Health. It never panned out as a cancer drug and was shelved until HIV came along, when the patent owner, Burroughs Wellcome (now GlaxoSmithKline), brushed off the dust and began studying it as an anti–HIV medicine. A 1986 clinical trial found phenomenal success, and America quickly revved itself into the first of what would be a series of overly optimistic assessments of our ability to quickly and easily end AIDS.

AZT did momentarily halt death rates, but that success proved unsustainable. The drug slowed HIV's progression in the body but couldn't maintain long-term control. Science stayed on the virus' trail, gradually adding new drugs to the treatment arsenal throughout the early 1990s. The turning point, however, came in 1996, when Dr. David Ho walked into the biennial International AIDS Conference—reconvening in Mexico City this August—and shocked the world by demonstrating his ability to bring patients back from the brink of death.

Ho had been among a handful of ambitious, young researchers who aggressively pursued HIV from the epidemic's onset. He was already credited with, among other things, establishing that saliva doesn't carry enough of the virus for it to be transmitted via kissing and, conversely, that HIV lives well in semen. In the mid-1980s, he was among the first to notice that a new HIV infection is usually accompanied by a brief period of flu-like symptoms, and much of his research from then on focused on how HIV behaves immediately after entering the body.

Conventional wisdom in the mid-1990s was that the virus sat dormant for years before launching its attack. Ho established that it actually engages the human body in a turf war from the beginning to the end—copying itself millions of times a day as it struggles to outpace the immune system. The take-away for Ho was that, contrary to treatment norms at the time, the immune system needs help before patients start getting sick, at which point the body is already losing the fight.

He matched the existing AIDS meds with a new class of drugs called protease inhibitors and bombarded the immune system with an intensive regimen. HIV couldn't mutate fast enough to get around this "combination therapy," so the immune system could catch up with it and beat patients' viral loads down to immeasurably small numbers. After 15 years of steadily increasing death rates, the numbers fell by 21 percent in a single year. By 1998, mortality had dropped by an astounding 70 percent.

It was morning in America. *Time* magazine named Ho its 1996 Man of the Year. The *New York Times Magazine* ran a cover story titled, "When Plagues End." *The Wall Street Journal, Newsweek*, and others chimed in with similar speculation about the end of AIDS. In a sign of just how nonchalant we became, it wasn't long before the treatment Ho dreamed up became popularly known as the "AIDS cocktail"—an odd moniker for something that's far more akin to a lifelong chemotherapy treatment than happy hour. Drug company ads featuring buff men rock climbing and mountain biking proliferated—people with AIDS, once pariahs, got modeling opportunities.

The much-touted magical turnaround was, however, uneven from its start. The drugs are extremely expensive, today costing as much as $20,000 for a year's treatment, not counting all of the auxiliary care and meds that are needed to stay healthy. Moreover, making them work well means having medical providers schooled in a rapidly changing, cutting-edge treatment science. Black Americans are less likely to have either of these resources, and the racial differential in AIDS death rates reflects that fact. Indeed, the death rate for 1996 marked two huge turning points in the epidemic: Not only was it the first year in which fewer people died than the year before, it was also the first year in which more blacks died than whites. By 2004, nearly twice as many blacks as whites died from AIDS.

All signs point to that disparity growing, in part because the number of African Americans infected is likely higher than we know, particularly in the South. The CDC has tracked the epidemic by counting the number of people who test positive each year and extrapolating from that an estimate of the total number infected. Until now, researchers haven't been able to differentiate between an infection that happened three months ago and three years ago –which means they can't tell how fast or slow the virus is spreading, or where and among whom. At press time, however, the CDC was preparing to release the results of a closely guarded study that deploys new technology to determine how long ago a newly diagnosed infection took place. The study is expected to raise the agency's estimate for the size of the epidemic by as much as half, a growth driven by infections among African Americans.

The million-dollar question, of course, is *why* blacks are so much more likely to both get infected with and die from HIV.

The theories are manifold, ranging from biology to public-policy failures. On the policy end of things, one villain is clearly the prison system. One of the many ways in which the massive forced migration of black men in and out of state and federal lockup destroys communities is through spreading disease. "It's definitely in there," says Tracy of the sex he saw in prison. "And ain't no condoms." Just two states allow condoms behind bars, virtually ensuring the spread of infectious diseases. Forward-thinking researchers have begun tracking how that reverberates into the broader community, perhaps explaining why two-thirds of new infections are logged among black women.

Regardless of what goes on inside prisons, the act of churning so many men in and out of black neighborhoods is itself a disease vector. Research shows that black women are more likely than women of other races to be serial monogamists, cycling through relationships with a small circle of men who come in and out of their lives—which means once one person in that circle gets infected, the virus spreads through it like brush fire. Black Americans with HIV/AIDS are also far less likely to be in treatment than their white peers—and because effective treatment lowers the amount of HIV in an infected person's blood, black people are therefore more likely to pass on the virus during unprotected sex.

And so the widespread existence of untreated HIV inside small, overlapping black sexual networks makes someone inside that network all the more likely to encounter it, meaning the same decision about whether to have unprotected sex involves far greater stakes. It's an insidious, self-reinforcing loop.

WHATEVER IS CAUSING the racial disparity in infection rates, it is ultimately going to collapse the system we built to make AIDS care accessible in the United States. The fast-growing African American epidemic is both heavily reliant upon the public-care system and deeply Southern. Two-thirds of black people getting AIDS care pay for it with public insurance. And nowhere are the racial disparities in who's getting infected more stark than in the South. South Carolina's epidemic is 74 percent black. North Carolina's is 68 percent. Alabama's is 64 percent. These states have been utterly unable to meet the demand those numbers reflect.

When I met Tracy in 2005, Alabama was experiencing what everyone hoped would be a wake-up call. The state-run program that makes AIDS drugs affordable to uninsured patients had a waiting list of more than 600 people. The previous year, the national total for people waiting for treatment had hit an all-time high, at just over 1,600. So, in what has been a decades-long pattern of piecemeal solutions to AIDS, the feds and the state patched together emergency funding and cleared Alabama's list.

By 2006, AIDS–funding problems were cropping up elsewhere in the region. South Carolina had replaced Alabama as the crisis of the moment. That November, after months of warnings from AIDS service providers around the state, the health department confirmed everyone's fears: Three people had died while waiting for access to the AIDS Drug Assistance Program, known as ADAP; a fourth died less than a month later. South Carolina's waiting list was finally cleared last summer, but the state has long been a standout offender in turning away people who can't afford AIDS medications. The state's waiting list has averaged just over 300 people since the summer of 2002, giving it the second-worst record in the country, behind neighboring North Carolina.

When AZT hit the market in 1987, its whopping price tag of $10,000 for a year's treatment spurred AIDS activists to storm the stock exchange and blockade the Food and Drug Administration, demanding the price come down. Congress responded by handing out a series of small, one-time grants to states and cities to subsidize the price of AZT. The 1990 Ryan White CARE Act finally created what was to be a soup-to-nuts response, setting up a Byzantine formula to distribute money to cities and states based on the intensity of their individual epidemics. Local health departments spend the federal money on a range of services needed to keep people healthy, including ADAP.

The CARE Act has been remarkably successful in keeping low-income Americans with HIV/AIDS alive. Medicaid and Medicare are the nation's largest payers for AIDS treatment, but ADAP fills the growing gap between those poor enough to qualify for public insurance and those with robust enough private insurance to afford the high-end medical care an HIV infection demands. However, as the legislation's name implies—it's the Comprehensive AIDS Resources *Emergency* Act—lawmakers never understood it as a permanent entity that would require ongoing and increasing support.

David Ho's treatment revolution turned the AIDS–care safety net from a hospice program into one that subsidizes exorbitantly expensive long-term treatment. Drug costs for people enrolled in ADAP reached an estimated $1.2 billion last year. That level of spending has simply proven unsustainable, particularly in Southern states, which are home to more than a third of ADAP clients. The South's budget troubles are partially due to the fact that Southern state legislatures don't chip in to support the program as much as those in the Northeast and West, leaving the health departments more heavily dependent upon federal money. Southern AIDS activists insist, however, that Washington shares some blame because the CARE Act's complicated funding formula has for years been weighted in favor of the cities and states with older epidemics.

But no matter how Congress divides the money, the reality is that there's just not enough to go around. Even as ADAP has grown exponentially, the federal contribution to it has either remained flat or, as it did last year, declined. Similarly, the CARE Act has not seen a meaningful funding increase since 2003, despite the fact that the epidemic hit a record high in 2005 and has grown by anywhere from 40,000 to 60,000 infections a year since then. And according to the federal agency that administers the CARE Act, nearly half of those people will turn to the program for help. Whether they'll find it depends on where they live.

The system has survived thus far on a series of last-minute rescues. When waiting lists hit their peak in 2004, the White House shepherded through Congress a one-time infusion of cash to 10 states with backlogs. In 2006, Congress gave the program another one-time shot in the arm. Several states have also been able to shift drug costs into the expanded Medicare program. And some Southern states, most notably South Carolina, have finally cobbled together their own AIDS–care budgets. By September 2007 there were, for the first time, no waiting lists. Few expect that victory to survive the fiscal year, however.

The recurring funding shortages are owed in part to the same ideological nickel-and-diming that's undermined a wide range of domestic programs in the Bush era. But it is also clear that America has never come to grips with the fact that AIDS demands a comprehensive, ongoing public-health commitment rather than finger-in-the-dam, emergency measures. Here's a telling fact: The U.S. has never had an overarching national plan for responding to AIDS, something that we make a prerequisite for any poorer country seeking foreign aid to deal with its own epidemic.

THE DISARRAY CAUSED by this lack of planning reaches past ADAP, or even the broader net of HIV/AIDS treatment and care. Last spring, CDC director Julie Gerberding convened what the agency billed as a historic meeting of African American community leaders to enlist them in launching a new, comprehensive prevention push. Gerberding implored a crowd that ranged from Urban League executives to rap star Ludacris' mom to make HIV a priority. "You can't solve big problems with small investments," Gerberding said wisely. "You need big investments to solve big problems." She vowed to take the same message to Congress.

No one listened. The CDC's HIV–prevention budget has never topped $800 million and has declined or remained flat every year this century. The only area of the prevention budget that's increased in recent years is that for testing, though even that money has actually come from moving cash out of other piles, according to the Community HIV/AIDS Mobilization Project.

The CDC has made testing the central plank of its prevention work. The agency cites studies that show roughly a quarter of all HIV–positive Americans don't know they are infected and that these undiagnosed cases are fueling the spread of the virus. So in 2006, the CDC changed its guidelines for hospitals and began recommending that every patient aged 13 to 64 be tested for HIV, rather than just those that report behaviors known to be particularly risky. It also streamlined the process, getting rid of a long-standing recommendation that clinicians provide counseling alongside testing. The change raises many difficult and uncomfortable questions. No one can argue with the goal of getting more people diagnosed, but is it enough to matter? It took Tracy 12 years to deal with his infection after he got diagnosed without counseling. And once hospitals identify the unknown hordes of HIV–positive patients, how will we provide them with treatment and care when the system is already overloaded?

Then again, maybe that's the catastrophic push we need to find a lasting solution to caring for people living with a disease that demands at least $12,000 per year in treatment to stave off death. The CDC's AIDS–prevention director, Kevin Fenton, warns, "The long-term costs of not diagnosing [infections] are going to be tremendous." It's only a question of whether we do it on the front end or, like the developing-world countries we look at with such pity, we do it after so many people are infected that the problem becomes unmanageable. Fenton put it best when he defended the testing push shortly after its rollout. "Whichever way you look at it, we're going to have to deal with this epidemic in real ways."

Another AIDS Casualty

David France

From *New York Magazine*

Dr. Ramon Torres was a hero on the front lines against the epidemic for over a decade. It was when the war began to be won that he got lost.

It WAS A frigid morning last December, and the disheveled man standing before Judge James Gibbons had made his way to the second floor of 100 Centre Street in a thin nylon windbreaker, ill-fitting designer jeans, and a pair of torn jackboots—something out of an old S&M catalogue—which he had accessorized with a wide leather cuff snapped on his wrist. At first he was trembling, as if from the cold. Then the trembling subsided, and his eyelids fell. Dr. Ramon A. "Gabriel" Torres, a near-legendary doctor in the fight against AIDS, had fallen asleep on his feet.

I remembered the first time I had seen him nod off in a crowded room. It was a decade ago, and Torres was the featured speaker at a meeting of top AIDS researchers to discuss a novel way to treat HIV-negative patients who suffered an accidental exposure—a needle stick or broken condom, or a night spent carelessly. At the time, Torres was the director of AIDS programs at St. Vincent's Medical Center. He was a visionary, responsible for turning a conservative Catholic clinic at the crossroads of the epidemic into a leading research facility, pioneering drug regimens that saved thousands of lives, and bringing AIDS care to homeless New Yorkers, the accomplishment for which he's best known.

Back then, I supposed that he must have been overcome by exhaustion. Shaken awake by applause, he walked to the microphone in his Armani suit and gave a presentation with all the gravitas befitting his reputation. But he made no sense whatsoever. His words were English, individually well formed. They just didn't seem to fit together.

When I mentioned this to a friend a day or two later, he said, "Oh, I know. Everybody knows."

What they knew was that Torres had begun his long romance with drugs. I have since seen him stumbling blurry-eyed and shirtless through the Chelsea night—once I saw him coming out of a notorious West Side drug emporium. There have been reports of drugged encounters in bathhouses, dance clubs, and sex Websites, then arrest after arrest.

Despite numerous trips to rehab, he had squandered his standing among AIDS clinicians and investigators, surrendered admitting privileges, been locked out of his West 23rd Street practice, lost his Chelsea apartment and Miami Beach condo, watched his Fire Island home collapse into foreclosure. He'd accumulated ten criminal charges, some of them felonies stemming from, among other accusations, allegations that he saw patients while his license was temporarily suspended for practicing while high. The first of his trials is scheduled to begin next week. If convicted on all of them, he technically could get as much as 31 years in prison, although somewhere between two and seven years is much more likely.

On the morning he dozed before Judge Gibbons, a simultaneous hearing was taking place in absentia to strip him of his medical license permanently.

"I can't be in two places at one time," Torres had whispered to me when he first arrived in court. He showed me a pink slip of paper from the Office of Professional Medical Conduct, then folded it back into his front pocket vacantly. It was the only thing he carried. "I already informed them by phone, fax, and letter that this is going on. But they wouldn't change the date."

Torres is one of the untold casualties of the epidemic's aftershocks. In the decade since AIDS moved from a mostly deadly plague to a largely manageable condition, a surprising number of the frontline veterans of the most difficult years in the fight against the disease have seemed to lose their bearings. Many health-care professionals talk today of feelings of emptiness and disillusionment in the wake of the epidemic's taming. Some have moved out of the field altogether. For others, drug addiction replaced drug research. Dr. Scott Hitt, the chairman of Bill Clinton's AIDS advisory commission who died of cancer in November, was stripped of his license for drug possession and admitted to inappropriate contact with two patients. A few years earlier, Jeffrey Wallach, a city clinician with a huge AIDS practice, died of an apparent overdose after years of abusing steroids and other drugs. "I could probably name 50 other docs off the top of my head who were not as well known but were certainly as much on the front lines who have had all different kinds of issues and problems," says Ken Fornataro, the executive director of AIDS Treatment Data Network, "and that's just in New York."

There is no way to know statistically if these stories are more prevalent among AIDS doctors than, say, oncologists. The playwright and activist Larry Kramer, for one, is critical of suggestions that AIDS pioneers have misbehaved disproportionately. But he admits he has heard anecdotes of doctors who made superhuman contributions during the darkest years of AIDS only to fall apart after 1996. "What do they do between 1985 and

1996?" Kramer says. "Huh? That's eleven years—eleven fucking years. If you're a doctor in the midst of all of that, and you've got hundreds of patients, and every one of them is facing death and is terrified, of course you're going to crack up. You wouldn't be a human being if you didn't."

Spencer Cox, an ACT UP veteran who founded a think tank called the Medius Institute for Gay Men's Health, suggests that anybody who lived through the worst of the AIDS crisis has lasting trauma and tends to suffer elevated levels of drug problems, starting later in life. "These aren't people who were ticking time bombs to begin with and then skidded off the road. They're our best and brightest. I can't tell you how many terrific, smart, hardworking, amazing people I know hit middle age and just lost it," he says.

As Torres stood sleeping before Judge Gibbons, court clerks thumbed through paperwork frantically. Finally, the judge spoke, and Torres lifted his head. "I see there is an open bench warrant," Judge Gibbons said finally. It turned out Torres had missed a court date on unrelated charges, one involving an alleged assault on a neighbor in his old Chelsea apartment and another alleging drug possession. Unbeknownst to him, a warrant for his arrest had been issued in October.

His attorney, Barry Agulnick, protested to the judge. "He believed that that case had been dismissed. Why would he skip?"

"The problem could be," Gibbons interrupted, "that due to a drug habit, he's amassing cases so fast he cannot keep track of them."

He ordered Torres—"or Dr. Torres, if you indeed are a doctor"—held on $5,000 bail. It was a sum that Torres couldn't produce. So he was handcuffed and led to the Tombs, where he would spend the next week.

"He's hit the bottom," said Agulnick. "Some guys catch a break every once in a while. With Torres, it's never."

The next week, Agulnick quit the case; he hadn't been paid in months.

AIDS wasn't yet on the horizon when Gabriel Torres set his sights on medicine. The oldest son of a sugarcane farmhand from Ponce, in southern Puerto Rico, Torres was lured to NYU in 1976 with a large financial-aid package to become the first member of his family to earn a degree. He went to Columbia University College of Physicians and Surgeons as a National Health Service Corps scholar, which requires young doctors to spend a number of years working with underserved populations in exchange for full tuition. Diabetes and nephrology were in his plans, not infectious diseases.

That changed in 1983, the year he arrived at St. Vincent's to participate in a training rotation. As a gay man, he'd heard about the new scourge. But he was too deep in his books to notice the burgeoning human toll. By that point, over 1,000 people had died of what would come to be called AIDS, yet it was still possible to live in New York and be unaware that the city was the new pandemic's epicenter.

Torres's eyes were opened when he entered the intensive-care unit on one of his first rounds. Young gay men occupied eight of the nine beds. Breathing tubes animated their lungs, which were wracked by *Pneumocystis carinii* pneumonia, a previously rare affliction that the Centers for Disease Control was monitoring as part of a mysterious new outbreak. Kneeling next to one of the beds, the frantic mother of a comatose Venezuelan patient was screaming at the boyfriend she'd just learned her son had, while banging her forehead against the floor.

Throughout the hospital were other signs of the coming plague. The emergency room swelled with patients for whom there were no treatments, Torres said, with opportunistic infections so rare they didn't appear in modern textbooks. "All around the hospital," Torres says, "you saw Kaposi's sarcoma and vascular dermatosis, a growth that turns your skin violaceous—it looks like you have grapes growing out of your skin, pendulous grapes; I mean your body is covered entirely with it."

One man came in with a strange complaint: He looked and felt perfectly healthy, except that his ears were filled with the sound of a helicopter rotor—a symptom, it turned out, of AIDS-related cryptococcal meningitis, which produced intense pressure on his spinal fluids. "We thought he was malingering, but he was dead in a week," he says. "I still remember his name."

At the time, some city hospitals were refusing AIDS patients, shipping them instead to larger teaching facilities. Those that did accept patients often embraced draconian isolation policies. Back then I was working at the New York *Native,* the city's gay newspaper, fielding calls from people stranded in hospital rooms where no doctors visited them and food trays were left outside the door—patients who were too weak to leave their own beds were sometimes left in their own waste. No hospital received more bitter complaints for more years than St. Vincent's. "It was so completely insulting that this was happening in the Village, in the epicenter of gay life and the epidemic," says Jim Hubbard, the co-founder of the ACT UP Oral History Project. "People would stream out of the ACT UP meeting and go and demonstrate at the hospital right then, because it was so awful."

In this environment, it was also rare for medical students to set their sights on AIDS. Most doctors were terrified about contamination. Dr. Anthony Fauci, today the nation's highest AIDS official, darkly speculated that transmission might occur otherwise than through bodily fluids. As a result, some doctors wrapped themselves in spacesuitlike protective gear for examining AIDS patients. Others refused to give medical attention altogether. A 1987 survey of doctors in training at New York City hospitals found that a quarter believed it was ethically acceptable to refuse treatment to an AIDS patient. It didn't get much better over the next few years. As recently as 1990, when a million Americans were living with the virus and 100,000 were already dead, half of all general practitioners said they wouldn't treat people suffering from the disease, given the chance.

That left the job to a small group of extremely young doctors, mostly women and social-justice types or gay men and lesbians. Says Ronald Bayer, a Columbia professor of public health who has compiled an oral history of AIDS physicians, *AIDS Doctors: Voices From the Epidemic,* "Here was a moment when only the avant-garde did AIDS, and they were excoriated by their colleagues."

Among them, an "atmosphere of cowboy medicine" developed, Dr. Abigail Zuger, at the time a resident at Bellevue, said in Bayer's book. Dr. Joseph Sonnabend—one of the most influential experts on the epidemic, co-founder of the groups that became amfar and the AIDS Community Research Initiative of America as well as a number of other national organizations—personally smuggled pharmaceuticals through Customs that the FDA had banned. "I can't even begin to tell you what it was like," he says. "The unbelievable was normal—it's hard to conceive. It was like a state of siege, there was that sort of energy and hysteria."

Torres fulfilled his obligations to the National Health Service Corps by taking a posting at the Wards Island Men's Shelter, which St. Vincent's ran under contract to the city. While there, the young doctor published studies in prestigious medical journals, mainly focusing on AIDS among marginalized New Yorkers. He conducted the nation's first HIV-prevalence survey among homeless men, for instance, revealing the startling fact that 62 percent carried the virus—an early indicator that AIDS had jumped the boundaries of the gay community. Partly on the basis of that study, which made headlines in the *New York Times* in 1989, he was offered the top AIDS job at St. Vincent's in 1990.

In truth, he had no competition. "Nobody wanted the job," Torres tells me. At the time, the hospital's AIDS office was in a storage room on the ground floor of the O'Toole Building, across Seventh Avenue from the hospital, according to Mike Barr, then a staff member. By all accounts, Torres attacked the challenge with unequaled imagination. St. Vincent's had never been a significant research hospital, but Torres quickly saw a different way to develop the clinic. He began enrolling his patients in cutting-edge pharmaceutical trials, which not only gained them access to promising treatments but also produced an independent income stream for his clinic, at a time when drug companies were paying a lot for access to patients.

At its peak, the clinic had 40 studies running, worth perhaps hundreds of millions of dollars a year. "We had so much money that, quite frankly, it was hard to spend it fast enough," says Mary Catherine George, the research administrator at the clinic. But spend it they did. The staff grew to include twenty nurse practitioners and fourteen full-time physicians, including psychiatrists and oncologists. They were investigating everything from ways to keep patients from getting pneumonias to the efficacy of the so-called D-drugs, ddI and ddC. St. Vincent's joined vaccine trials, drug-"cocktail" trials, and studies of salvage therapies for people with multiple drug resistance. Torres became one of the world's experts on the ways HIV medications alter body shapes of patients and the dual problems of HIV and TB infections, especially among transsexuals and the homeless, who remained his passion.

In fact, it was his work among New York's most-forgotten communities that set Torres apart from other AIDS doctors. He forged outreach programs to illegal immigrants, intravenous-drug users, transgender patients, and even male prostitutes. This often put him at odds with hospital directors and the Archdiocese. Noel George, who was Torres's senior research nurse for many of those years, says, "The hospital kept blocking research because they didn't want condoms mentioned in the consent form." When Torres wanted to conduct a study of treating people after inadvertent exposures, the hospital refused, arguing that it seemed to be promoting unsafe sex. "I was pushing the envelope," Torres admits. "They were very uncomfortable about some of the things we were doing."

But he was given unusual leeway because AIDS, thanks to New York State reimbursement levels, was exceedingly profitable for St. Vincent's. On peak days, AIDS patients filled 120 beds, more than a third of the hospital's overall capacity, with even more waiting in the hallways, according to Torres. "There was just mayhem. Gurneys everywhere, people with IVs in chairs, IVs running out of fluid. A nursing shortage. I mean those days were absolute craziness."

There also was a staggering amount of suffering and death. Despite their efforts, every year close to a third of St. Vincent's AIDS patients passed away.

Instead of being disheartened, Torres sacrificed everything for the clinic and his patients. Increasingly in demand as a public speaker, he folded his honoraria back into the operating budget. He hardly took vacations, or even a weekend away. "It was more stressful to try to go away than to stay and work," he tells me. "Not only did I have a lot of patients in the hospital, but a lot of them were my friends. I couldn't leave them."

Torres's ingenuity and passion for the work made him a kind of cult figure. I attended a medical conference once where he stirred up an ovation just by walking into the room. A small number of top AIDS doctors enjoyed similar acclaim. Paul Volberding, who directed the San Francisco General AIDS clinic and is a global leader in AIDS research and care, keeps a letter that reached his office mailbox from England though it was addressed simply to "Dr. Paul, San Francisco."

But even among his peers, Torres stood out. "There was no bigger star," says Dr. Victoria Sharp, director of AIDS programs at St. Luke's–Roosevelt. "The thing about Gabe was, he went to Columbia. He published. He was gorgeous—drop-dead gorgeous. And he was so humble. I mean, there was nothing missing."

Or so it seemed.

Until the mid-nineties, Torres was as sober as one of the nuns who float through the halls at St. Vincent's. He says he still doesn't drink; wine gives him a headache. He claims to have smoked exactly two joints in his life, and has no desire to try again. But in 1994 or 1995, one of his friends offered him Special K, or ketamine, a horse tranquilizer then popular as a club drug. He experimented with it for a while. It was, Torres says, the perfect drug for a hopeless epidemic. "You just wanted to deaden yourself," he says. "K anesthetizes the pain." But the minute he felt the drug impeding his life, he declared it off-limits. Besides, there was much to celebrate all of a sudden. Beginning in 1996, new drug regimens Torres helped bring about abruptly changed the course of AIDS, ushering in the first good news in the fifteen-year epidemic. Almost overnight, people grew healthier and the daily inpatient population at St. Vincent's dropped from 120 to 70, then 40, then fewer.

Soon, friends say, Torres was turning to crystal. It was a time when the drug—methamphetamine, long popular as working-class speed, with a following in rural America —was beginning to claim a foothold among urban gay men. Most weren't reckless kids. "The biggest meth demographic is gay men who survived AIDS and are now in their forties," says Peter Staley, an HIV-positive recovering addict. "I've always called it the perfect midlife-crisis drug." Berkeley, California–based psychotherapist Walt Odets calls meth use an understandable reaction to the severe and repeated losses from the worst plague years. "This didn't have some kind of clean ending," he says. "I read a quote from Mike Nichols, the director, who said once, 'That's all blood under the bridge.' That's what AIDS is like."

The drug quickly had Torres in a bind. "He was going through several thousand dollars a week on meth," according to Darren Allumier, who was Torres's boyfriend for ten years. "He's always had this amazing ability to—what's it called?—hold his liquor and drugs and still function normally. But at home, he was the complete opposite." Allumier narrates a behind-the-scenes fall into addiction marked by sleeplessness, violence, and repeat calls to 911. It first came to a head one Friday afternoon when the two were leaving for Fire Island. The trip seemed to cause Torres great anxiety, stirring up insecurities about his impact as a doctor. He began to berate himself. "He took a fistful of keys and began pounding himself on the head and neck and back until he was all bloody," Allumier says. According to both men, violence between them escalated over the following months, culminating in a final breakup in the spring of 1998, followed by endless ad hominems and, briefly, a charge of attempted murder.

"The foundation under him crumbled" is how Allumier sees Torres's drug use. But Torres spins it in a more positive light. "I always say the crystal was for celebration, not to take care of my pain or whatever," he says. "I was celebrating the fact that now everyone was living and not dying. It seemed like a reason to celebrate, and crystal was a perfect drug for that. You've got all this energy. You stay up. You dance." He adds, "You wanted to feel alive."

Simultaneously, the horizon for his AIDS clinic began to look bleak. Fewer admissions meant he was no longer the hospital's rainmaker. And for a long time after the protease revolution, few new drugs entered into research. "Suddenly, we had no grant money, no research to pursue," says Mary Catherine George. "We went off a cliff."

The hospital administration began dismantling Torres's program, relocating his physicians to other departments and putting the operation on a shorter financial leash. Similar constrictions were happening in other hospitals. But for Torres, it was a destabilizing blow. "I felt totally defeated," he says. "It was tearing me apart."

He responded with more "celebrations." "It became the only way of escaping all this craziness," he says. An acquaintance—a physician's assistant who specializes in AIDS—watched mutely as Torres slid from losing his presentation materials at a medical conference, to appearing wasted at a gay bathhouse, to wearing sunglasses in his own office, rocking like a junkie. "I've been in recovery now for eighteen years," says the acquaintance. "I would see doctors and other health-care providers who I knew at some gay event like the Black Party. They'd all be higher than God. There was part of me that in one respect was almost envious. I would say to my husband, how can these guys do it? How can they do drugs and still have a successful practice? And then, of course, they didn't. It eventually caught up."

Many leading AIDS physicians acknowledge the trend among some doctors, which they consider understandable, given the circumstances. "If what happened to Gabriel is one response, there are of course many who responded in other ways," says Sonnabend, who today is retired in London and, by his own assessment, mostly broke and lonely but untouched by addiction, though he has buried all but one of his ex-lovers and most of his friends. "How can I be unaffected by all of that? How the hell can I be? How is it possible? I've been quite hurt." Dr. Donna Futterman, a veteran expert in adolescent AIDS at Montefiore Hospital, agrees. "If I was a gay man instead of a gay woman back then," she says, "I would have been dead in five years."

Doctors were not the only surprise casualties of the protease era. Many heads of AIDS groups and activists have tumbled into addiction, disillusionment, career crisis, or worse. After years of vigilance, many have recently contracted HIV, says the Medius Institute's Cox. "Having worked in HIV seems to be a risk for recent HIV infection," he says.

"Of course these people got lost—I almost got lost," says Rodger McFarlane, the first executive director of GMHC (at age 26), who went on to found and run some of the city's leading AIDS agencies. "Nobody talks about it, but it was the most fun I ever had in my life. I never got out of bed with so much energy and so sure of what I needed to do and surrounded by the coolest people, who became respected in our fields. It's like wartime. When are the relationships so immediate, when are the stakes so high? When do you see the impact you as an individual can have and see radical change made? I mean, it was horrible. It was outrageous. And it seemed to take years. But look what we did!

It's historic shit. You don't have that crack again. You bet these people got lost when they're not that person anymore. I'm not talking about ego. You're the hot shit in the biggest disease, and then treatment becomes available, and then what? Now you go to clinic every day and write prescriptions?"

In early 1998, at the suggestion of his colleague Dr. David Ho of the Aaron Diamond AIDS Research Center, Torres agreed to meet with a wealthy entrepreneur named Bernie Salick, who planned to finance a flashy, holistic AIDS center on Irving Place, in a facility designed by Gwathmey Siegel & Associates. Salick offered him a star's position there, more than doubling his salary to over $350,000—an enormous sum for someone who grew up as poor as Torres had.

The first thing Torres did after he took the job was buy a house in the Pines, and an apartment in Miami Beach—in cash. Every Friday during that first winter, he flew to Florida to party with a new group of friends, a life he'd never even dreamed of attaining. "I was making more money than I'd ever made and spending more than I'd ever spent," he says. He almost never made it back to work by Monday morning. He sometimes missed Tuesday as well. "He would call me and say, 'I'm in the tunnel,'" remembers Mary Catherine George, who followed Torres to the Salick facility. "I'd say, 'Well, get the hell out of the tunnel and get into this office. There are patients waiting for you since yesterday.'"

In the middle of this slide, Torres's mother lost her long battle with cancer in 2000. Her death sent him into a Niagara of grief, his friends say. "I was flatlines," Torres agrees, crying intensely years later. "I was emotionally dead. I didn't have aspirations to do much of anything."

Thereafter, people all over the city began to notice that he was falling apart. At a GMHC dinner at the Waldorf featuring Lainie Kazan, according to a witness, his head fell comically into his dinner plate before friends dragged him outside. Eventually, the rumors got so bad that Brian Saltzman, one of his partners, confronted his friend. "I said, 'I don't know what's going on. I haven't seen you impaired, but there are these allegations. If there is anything going on, I suggest you call the OPMC,'" Saltzman remembers, referring to the Office of Professional Medical Conduct. "He absolutely denied there was any problem."

In an unrelated twist, the posh private practice was going bust anyway. A third partner, Todd Yancey, had been accused of inappropriate sexual contact with a few patients, one of whom committed suicide—he reportedly left a long note blaming Yancey for his depression. The family threatened legal action. Yancey agreed to retire his license, acknowledging he could not defend himself against the charges, and Bernard Salick shuttered the practice soon thereafter.

Next, both Saltzman and Torres headed to Beth Israel. But Torres's downward spiral continued. One lunch break, he fell asleep in his car—for three hours—and missed a string of appointments, resulting in a suspension for suspected drug use (he takes issue with this characterization, saying that his "somnolence" was owed to "overusing Benadryl" and that he hadn't used crystal for several days before the incident). Following evaluation at Marworth, a Pennsylvania rehab facility, he was allowed to return on the condition that he submit to random urine tests, but he tested positive five weeks later. He remained on medical leave from the hospital until he resigned on October 11, 2001.

He didn't quit using, though. Instead, he applied for a number of jobs, including at St. Luke's–Roosevelt with his old friend Dr. Victoria Sharp. She recalls the day he showed up for an interview. "My secretary said, 'My God, this guy looks like he's on drugs.' He looked terrible." After receiving him in her office, Sharp expressed concern without mincing words. He rebuffed her. "Quite frankly," he tells me, "I didn't think it was any of her business." She later called a meeting of other top AIDS experts at the bar at the Carlyle to discuss an intervention, but nothing seems to have been done. Later, Torres was offered the job of medical director at Housing Works, the agency for homeless

New Yorkers with HIV. At the time, I was on the board of directors. In a bitter fight with the co-founder, Keith Cylar, I argued
against putting Torres in a position where lives depended upon
him unless he was demonstrably rehabilitated. The offer was
rescinded.

Finding himself unemployable, Torres set himself up in
private practice in Chelsea, putting a drug-using administrator
in charge of running the office and a transgender woman at the
front desk. He never brought in enough money to make payroll.
"I was able to keep it going by refinancing my Fire Island house
every six months or so," he says.

But there was still further to fall. In early 2004, Torres took
himself to Miami for a circuit party, a big event on the gay social
calendar. As he boarded his return flight the following Monday
morning, agents found a crystal pipe in the pocket of his bomber
jacket. "It belonged to this trick I picked up," he told a friend.
"It wasn't even mine." They threw him in jail until he could post
bail. He was to return in a few months for a court appearance
but missed the date by two days. "That's Gabriel," says his closest
friend, Paul Shelby, a massage therapist. "If there's a plane to
catch, he's going to miss it."

When he finally appeared, the judge angrily dispatched him
to a court-ordered residential rehab program for three months,
leaving his patients stranded.

Meanwhile, back in New York, his office manager—an
Israeli citizen named Joseph Kassous—apparently cleared out his
personal and corporate checking accounts; siphoned $400,000
more from Torres's good friend and patient, Baroness Rocio
Urquijo of Spain; sold or gave away scores of forged Percocet
prescriptions; and jumped bail after the police caught up with
him (he's still at large and believed to be in Mexico). Besides
bankrupting Torres, the events touched off an investigation by
the attorney general's office into his prescribing patterns. "My
name was found on bottles in all sorts of people's houses—drug

dealers, people who were arrested—all forged," Torres says. "They came down on me like an earthquake after Joseph."

"It was like something out of *Les Miz*," says Barry Agulnick, who represented him in the investigation. "There is one particular investigator who has been after him for years."

Ultimately, the investigation came to a close without charges against Torres, but not before the Office of Professional Medical Conduct opened its own probe. More than a year ago, it alleged that he had practiced medicine while intoxicated. It also alleged that he had misrepresented his history of administrative punishments on job applications, a serious violation of ethical code. Beginning on December 21, 2006, his license was suspended for at least twelve months.

Subsequently, he lost his Chelsea rental apartment following a protracted dispute with his landlord, neighbors, and city officials over his dogs (he was raising litters of boxer puppies in his tiny studio, where the floor was piled with feces). Last May, following a physical altercation with a neighbor over the matter, he was arrested and charged with third-degree assault. When he was frisked, police allegedly found a bag filled with powder. "It's crystal meth, my friend, give it to me," Torres reportedly demanded. Those charges are still outstanding.

Finally, last August, he was arrested in his office for practicing medicine while on suspension, a charge that involves multiple felonies, including grand larceny. Detectives searching his pockets say they found another envelope of crystal. He has entered not-guilty pleas on all counts, according to Darius Wadia, his new court-appointed attorney.

The total collapse of Gabriel Torres's life and career has distressed the few people in the AIDS Establishment aware of his plight. "It's just one of the biggest tragedies I've ever seen. This is a guy who had absolutely everything going for him," says John Grimaldi, a psychiatrist who worked for Torres at St. Vincent's and is now in practice in Memphis. "All of his colleagues are completely and totally heartbroken about this."

Jonathan Tobin, who undertook important AIDS research with Torres as head of New York's Clinical Directors Network, agrees. "Many people are alive because of him," he says, "and many others died with a greater sense of peace and dignity because of him. I hope in his time of suffering people will come to his assistance with the same selflessness."

The problem is, nobody knows how to help, or even how to reach him. "I would do anything I could to help him," says Sharp. "I just don't know what to do."

Last fall, as his case percolated through the courts, Torres kept a low profile at his Fire Island home, which he had been trying to sell in order to stave off foreclosure. He lived there on and off, despite having no electricity or insulation, until mid-January, when a cold snap exploded twenty pipes throughout the house. (It has since sold for less than he owed.) He returned to New York with his remaining dog, a boxer named Usmail, a reference to the Puerto Rican fairy tale in which a postage stamp is misread as a proper name. To support himself, Torres was selling his sizable art collection a piece at a time over Craigslist; he has also sold his bed, among other furniture. Finally, he had to give up the dog to an agency for adoption.

Torres at first bunked in with his current boyfriend at an SRO in Times Square, until guards there blacklisted him. With no options left, he went to a city agency, which found him a strict SRO on the Upper West Side—through a program geared for homeless people with HIV.

It seems Torres had fallen victim to the virus in more ways than one. He has been HIV-positive since 2002.

"I was infected by my last boyfriend—it was conscious," he explained to me awkwardly during a lengthy interview right before Christmas. "Well, not conscious. He was positive and I was negative and we were having unsafe sex." Was that because he was high on crystal at the time? I wondered. "We were both sober," he replied. "There is no one reason for every infection."

"What was the unsafe sex about, then?"

He answered uncertainly. "Love?"

When I saw him a few weeks later, Torres came to my apartment dressed in a fine but faded leather fetish jacket adorned with tight lacework and scores of silver grommets. His eyes looked clearer, and he spoke more lucidly about his situation than he had previously. It had been some time since he last did drugs—either several months, as he said, or several weeks, as seemed more accurate.

And he had a little money in his pocket. He had sold his computer, which allowed him to buy belated Christmas presents for his sister's children in New Jersey. The visit had put him in an upbeat mood. He had hope for his new lawyer and faith that he'll get probation, not jail time.

"I'm functional," he said proudly. But then he darkened. "I feel worse about the people I cared for. I feel that I've abandoned them."

Virtual Iraq: Using Simulation to Treat a New Generation of Traumatized Veterans.

Sue Halpern

from the *New Yorker*

The program uses sights, sounds, even smells to evoke, and subdue, painful memories.

IN NOVEMBER, 2004, when he was nineteen years old, a marine I'll call Travis Boyd found himself about to rush the roof of the tallest building in the northern end of Falluja in the midst of a firefight. Boyd, whose first assignment in Iraq was to the security detail at Abu Ghraib prison, had been patrolling the city with his thirteen-man infantry squad, rooting out insurgents and sleeping on the floors of abandoned houses, where they'd often have to remove dead bodies in order to lay out their bedrolls.

With Boyd in the lead, the marines ran up the building's four flights of stairs. When they reached the top, "the enemy cut loose at us with everything they had," he recalled. "Bullets were exploding like firecrackers all around us." Boyd paused and his team leader, whom he thought of as an older brother, ran past him to the far side of the building. Moments after he got there, he was shot dead. Within minutes, everyone else on the roof was wounded. "We had to crawl out of there," said Boyd, who was hit with shrapnel and suffered a concussion, earning a Purple Heart. "That was my worst day."

It is in the nature of soldiers to put emotions aside, and that is what Boyd did for three years. He "stayed on the line" with his squad and finished his tour of duty the following June, married his high-school girlfriend, and soon afterward began training for his second Iraq deployment, not thinking much about what he had seen or done during the first. Haditha, where he was sent in the fall of 2005, was calmer than Falluja. There were roadside bombs, but no direct attacks. Boyd was now a team leader, and he and his men patrolled the streets like police. When drivers did not respond to the soldiers' efforts to get them to stop, he said, "we'd have to light them up." He was there for seven months.

With one more year of service left on his commitment, and not enough time for a third deployment, Boyd was separated from his unit and assigned to fold towels and clean equipment at the fitness center of his Stateside base. It was a quiet, undemanding job, intended to allow him to decompress from combat. Instead, he was haunted by memories of Iraq. He couldn't sleep. His mind raced. He was edgy, guilt-racked, depressed. He could barely do his job.

"I'd avoid crowds, I'd avoid driving, I'd avoid going out at night," he told me the first time we spoke. "I'd avoid people who weren't infantry, the ones who hadn't been bleeding and dying and going weeks and months without showers and eating M.R.E.s. I'd have my wife drive me if I had to go off the base. A few times, I thought I saw a mortar in the road and reached for the steering wheel. I was always on alert, ready for anything to happen at any time."

Eventually, as part of a standard medical screening, Boyd was diagnosed as having chronic post-traumatic stress disorder. P.T.S.D., which in earlier conflicts was known as battle fatigue or

shell shock but is not exclusively war-related, has been an officially recognized medical condition since 1980, when it entered
the American Psychiatric Association's Diagnostic and Statistical
Manual of Mental Disorders. (In an earlier edition, it was called
"gross stress reaction.") P.T.S.D. is precipitated by a terrifying
event or situation—war, a car accident, rape, planes crashing
into the World Trade Center—and is characterized by nightmares, flashbacks, and intrusive and uncontrollable thoughts,
as well as by emotional detachment, numbness, jumpiness,
anger, and avoidance. Boyd's doctor prescribed medicine for
his insomnia and encouraged him to seek out psychotherapy,
telling him about an experimental treatment option called
Virtual Iraq, in which patients worked through their combat
trauma in a computer-simulated environment. The portal was a
head-mounted display (a helmet with a pair of video goggles),
earphones, a scent-producing machine, and a modified version
of Full Spectrum Warrior, a popular video game.

When Travis Boyd agreed to become a subject in the Virtual
Iraq clinical trial, in the spring of 2007, he became one of about
thirty-five active-duty and former members of the military to use
the program to treat their psychological wounds. Currently, the
Department of Defense is testing Virtual Iraq—one of three
virtual-reality programs it has funded for P.T.S.D. treatment,
and the only one aimed at "ground pounders" like Boyd—in
six locations, including the Naval Medical Center San Diego,
Walter Reed Army Medical Center, in Washington, D.C., and
Weill Cornell Medical College, in New York. According to a
recent study by the RAND Corporation, nearly twenty per cent
of Iraq and Afghanistan war veterans are suffering from P.T.S.D.
or major depression. Almost half won't seek treatment. If virtual-
reality exposure therapy proves to be clinically validated—only
preliminary results are available so far—it may be more than
another tool in the therapists' kit; it may encourage those in
need to seek help.

"Most P.T.S.D. therapies that we've seen don't seem to be working, so what's the harm in dedicating some money to R. & D. that might prove valuable?" Paul Rieckhoff, the executive director of Iraq and Afghanistan Veterans of America, said last November. In January, his group issued a lengthy report called "Mental Health Injuries: The Invisible Wounds of War," which cited research suggesting that "multiple tours and inadequate time at home between deployments increase rates of combat stress by 50%." Rieckhoff went on, "I'm not someone who responds to sitting with some guy, talking about my whole life. I'm going to go in and talk to some dude who doesn't understand my shit and talk about my mom? I'm the worst of that kind of guy. So V.R. therapy, maybe it will work. We're a video-game generation. It's what we grew up on. So maybe we'll respond to it."

Strictly speaking, using virtual reality to treat combat-related P.T.S.D. is not new. In 1997, more than twenty years after the Vietnam War ended, researchers in Atlanta unveiled Virtual Vietnam. It dropped viewers into one of two scenarios: a jungle clearing with a "hot" landing zone, or a Huey helicopter, its rotors whirring, its body casting a running shadow over rice paddies, a dense tropical forest, and a river. The graphics were fairly crude, and the therapist had a limited number of sights and sounds to manipulate, but Virtual Vietnam had the effect of putting old soldiers back in the thick of war. Ten combat veterans with long-term P.T.S.D. who had not responded to multiple interventions participated in a clinical trial of Virtual Vietnam, typically lasting a month or two. All of them showed significant signs of improvement, both directly after treatment and in a follow-up half a year later. (P.T.S.D. is assessed on a number of scales, some subjective and others based on the observation of the clinician.) As successful as it was, though, Virtual Vietnam didn't catch on. It was an experiment, and when the experiment was over the researchers moved on.

Like Virtual Vietnam, Virtual Iraq is a tool for doing what's known as prolonged-exposure therapy, which is sometimes called immersion therapy. It is a kind of cognitive-behavioral therapy, derived from Pavlov's classic work with dogs. Prolonged-exposure therapy, which falls under the rubric of C.B.T., is at once intuitively obvious and counterintuitive: it requires the patient to revisit and retell the story of the trauma over and over again and, through a psychological process called "habituation," rid it of its overwhelming power. The idea is to disconnect the memory from the reactions to the memory, so that although the memory of the traumatic event remains, the everyday things that can trigger fear and panic, such as trash blowing across the interstate or a car backfiring—what psychologists refer to as cues—are restored to insignificance. The trauma thus becomes a discrete event, not a constant, self-replicating, encompassing condition.

This process was explained to me by JoAnn Difede, the director of the Program for Anxiety and Traumatic Stress Studies at Weill Cornell, when I visited her in her office, last fall. Difede, a tough-minded New Yorker, began using virtual-reality exposure therapy with patients from the hospital's burn unit in the nineteen-nineties. She treated victims of September 11th with a program called Virtual W.T.C., which she designed with the creators of Virtual Vietnam, and is currently running a Virtual Iraq clinical trial as well as supervising therapists at other study sites.

Difede says that therapists have been slow to adopt exposure therapy, because they worry that it might be cruel to immerse a patient in a drowning pool of painful memories. It's a worry that, she believes, misses the point of the therapy. "If you suddenly become afraid of the staircase because you had to walk down twenty-five flights of stairs to get out of the World Trade Center, the stairs went from being neutral to being negative," Difede explained. "What we should be doing is extinguishing the cues associated with the stimuli, which should allow for a more complete remission, as well as mastery of the experience. It also should allow for greater emotional engagement. Because numbing and avoidance are symptoms of P.T.S.D., you're asking the person to do in treatment the very thing their mind is avoiding doing. That's quite a dilemma."

It's this dilemma that makes virtual reality especially attractive to clinical psychologists like Difede. Because the traumatic environment is produced in a computer graphics lab, and its elements are controlled by the therapist, virtual reality can nudge an imagination that is at once overactive and repressed. "Voilà, you're there!" Difede said. "You don't have to do any work. You don't have to engage in any mental effort. We'll do it for you. We'll bring you there and then, gradually, we'll let you get involved in the experience in sensory detail."

When Travis Boyd was first asked to consider enrolling in the Virtual Iraq clinical trial, he was hesitant. He had already decided not to talk to his division therapist, because "I didn't want to have it on my military record that I was crazy," he said. And he was a marine. "Infantry is supposed to be the toughest of the tough. Even though there was no punishment for going to therapy, it was looked down upon and seen as weak. But V.R. sounded pretty cool. They hook you up to a machine and you play around like a video game." Telling his buddies that he was going off to do V.R. was a lot easier than telling them he was seeing a shrink.

Before he was introduced to Virtual Iraq, the therapist asked him to close his eyes and talk about his wartime experiences. Without much prompting, he was back on the roof in Falluja, under fire, stalled at the top of the stairs, watching his friend and team leader run past him and die, and then he was dragging out his friend's body, looking at his messed-up face. When Boyd was finished, the doctor asked him to tell the story again. And, when he was finished that time, to tell it again. As he did, she asked him what he was smelling, and if the enemy was on the roof opposite or on the roof next door, and if there were planes overhead. She wanted to learn the details of his narrative and determine which moments were most troubling to him—she called them "hot spots"—and to figure out how she was going to use the sensory variables embedded in Virtual Iraq.

Boyd was introduced to the V.R. program in the third session. (There were twelve sessions in all, each about two hours long, over a period of six weeks.) Virtual-reality exposure therapy immerses the patient gradually; that first time Boyd just sat there with the V.R. gear on, looking at an Iraqi street scene, getting acquainted with the virtual world. Sound, which psychologists believe may stimulate memory more effectively than sight does, was added next, and, with it, touch. "I'm talking about the firefight and she turns on this vibrating thing so you feel like you're in a shaking building," Boyd said. "Each time she added something, like an I.E.D. going off, or a plane flying over, I'd become more emotional. We'd do it over and over, and it would become easier, and then she'd add something more and the same thing would happen. I'd talk for forty minutes about this one five-minute thing. When it's only visual, it's not really real— it's just a video game—but when the ground starts vibrating and you smell smoke and hear the AK-47 firing, it becomes very real. I'd be shaking. When it was over, I'd go home and cry."

The inventor of Virtual Iraq is Albert Rizzo, a clinical psychologist at the University of Southern California, who goes by the nickname Skip. Rizzo, who is fifty-three, has thinning black hair that's down to his shoulders when it's not pulled back in a ponytail, a stud earring, and a nose that looks like it has met a boot or two—he plays rugby. Rizzo rides a Harley 1200 Sportster ("It's not a girl's bike, no matter what anyone tells you"), plays blues harmonica (he taught himself a couple of years ago, in order to reduce stress when he was commuting daily in L.A. traffic), and has an affable, jeans-and-untucked-shirt way about him that is particularly noticeable when he walks through Walter Reed or the Naval Medical Center San Diego alongside his starched military counterparts. In 2003, not long after the United States invaded Iraq, Rizzo, who had been designing virtual-reality systems to diagnose attention deficits in children and memory problems in older adults, and was affiliated with the Institute for Creative Technologies, a U.S.C. offshoot that he likes to call "an unholy alliance between academia, Hollywood, and the military," had a hunch that, if the war went on for very long, its veterans were going to come home with serious emotional problems.

"I thought we should be on this so we don't have another Vietnam, with all these guys suffering from P.T.S.D.," he told me one day last fall at Walter Reed, before he was to give a presentation to senior military officers. "I was working on a talk about virtual reality, just sniffing around the Internet, and I saw this link for the video game Full Spectrum Warrior." The game had, in fact, originated as a training device that the Institute had developed for the Department of Defense. "I said, 'Oh, my God, that's Iraq!' It was instant. I thought we should take this game and run it in a head-mounted display right out of the box, for therapy."

Rizzo got in touch with Jarrell Pair, who had been the programmer on Virtual Vietnam, and convinced him to sign on to his as yet unfunded venture. By February, 2004, he and Pair had built a prototype of Virtual Iraq on a laptop, using a single street in an Iraqi market town which they had recycled from Full Spectrum Warrior. To this they added a few alternate realities that a therapist could insert with a keystroke—a change from day to night, for example, or a switch from a deserted street to one where burka-clad shoppers strolled down the sidewalk. "That was our demo," Rizzo said. "We applied for money and we got nuked. Then the Hoge article comes out and everything changes overnight."

The article to which Rizzo was referring was written by Charles Hoge and his colleagues in the Department of Psychiatry and Behavioral Sciences at Walter Reed and was published in the New England Journal of Medicine that summer. It was the first assessment of mental-health problems emerging from service in Iraq and Afghanistan, and even its conservative estimate—that around sixteen or seventeen per cent of those who fought in Iraq and eleven per cent who served in Afghanistan were suffering from P.T.S.D. symptoms (an estimate that four years later has been revised dramatically upward)—caught the public and the military by surprise. Then Rizzo got a call from somebody in the Office of Naval Research. "He says, 'I hear you've got a prototype of Full Spectrum Warrior for P.T.S.D.,' " Rizzo recalled. " 'We're going to try to get it funded.' "

The money came through in March, 2005, and by the next fall, right around the time that Travis Boyd was being deployed to police Haditha, the first patients were recruited to try it out.

Before Skip Rizzo started designing virtual-reality systems, he was a conventional clinical psychologist, schooled in a variety of therapeutic methods. Rizzo grew up just outside Hartford, attended the University of Hartford as an undergraduate, received a doctorate from Binghamton University, and did his internship at the V.A. hospital in Long Beach, California, not far from where he now lives. Then he took a job as a cognitive-rehabilitation therapist at a hospital in Costa Mesa, working with people who had suffered traumatic brain injuries. "A lot of young males are in that population," he said. "The high-risk-takers. The drunk drivers. Gang members—all of that. With that population, it was sometimes hard to motivate them to do the standard paper-and-pencil drill and practice routines. Then, in the early nineteen-nineties, Game Boys came on the scene, and it seemed to me that all my male clients, at every break, at every meal, had become Tetris warlords. It showed me that they were motivated to do game tasks, and that the more they did them the better they got, and it hit me that there could be a link between cognitive rehabilitation and virtual reality." Rizzo left his job, and accepted a postdoc at the Alzheimer Disease Research Center at U.S.C., where he began to design rudimentary virtual-reality systems with the help of programmers in the computer-science department. At the end of the postdoc, he moved to the engineering school at U.S.C. and started "building this stuff like crazy."

To make Virtual Iraq, Rizzo started with two basic scenarios: the market-town street scene and a Humvee moving along an Iraqi highway, where all the exit signs are in Arabic and the road cuts through sand dunes. Then he gave therapists a menu of ways—visual, aural, tactile, even olfactory—to customize them. At the click of a mouse, the therapist can put the patient in the driver's seat of the Humvee, in the passenger's seat, or in the turret behind a machine gun, and the vehicle moves at a speed determined by the patient. Maybe the gunner in the turret is wearing night-vision goggles—the landscape goes grainy and green. A sandstorm could be raging (the driver can turn on the windshield wipers and beat it back); a dog could be barking; the inside of the vehicle could be rank. Rizzo's idea is that giving the therapist so many options—dusk, midday; with snipers, without snipers; driving fast, creeping along; the sound of a single mortar, the sound of multiple mortars; the sound of people yelling in English or in Arabic—increases the likelihood of evoking the patient's actual experience, while engaging the patient on so many sensory levels that the immersion in the environment is nearly absolute.

"Tell me what you want me to add, anything," I overheard Rizzo asking a therapist at Walter Reed in February, a few days after she had completed a fourteen-session Virtual Iraq protocol in three months with the first soldier at the facility enrolled in the trial. (The patient didn't think he had got much better, though he was able to ride the subway again and no longer avoided large crowds.) "You're the one in the trenches hearing the stories. We'll keep evolving this to make it more relevant. What do you think about adding the smell of burning hair?"

Rizzo was sitting in a tiny, windowless room in front of a table ringed by a cloth skirt that partly hid the electrodes and other equipment that monitor a person's blood pressure, respiration, heart rate, and stress level during treatment, and were connected to two computers. He had flown in the night before to install the latest software upgrade, which he was introducing to the therapist, a slight young woman in her thirties.

"O.K.," Rizzo said as he clicked the computer mouse rapidly, "this is really cool." On the screen was the basic Virtual Iraq market scene: a few nearly empty vender stalls in the middle of a plaza and a row of small, ground-floor shops in dun-colored buildings lining the sidewalk. "You walk to the end of this street"—the sound of footsteps could be heard—"it's market east. Now, let's see if this works. Let me blow up this car." He clicked again and a small car about the size of a Toyota Corolla, which had been parked at the curb, burst into flames. "It's a good effect. Now, when you blow up the car, put in 'add stunned civilian.' One more thing—you have to learn where the R.P.G. guys are." He was referring to figures toting rocket-propelled grenades. "There's one here," he said, and on the screen there was another explosion. "Now we're going to head over there," he said, moving forward—more footsteps—toward a set of stairs. "Here's the deal with going up the stairs. You've got to hit it square on, otherwise you'll get caught up in the collision barrier. It just breaks the presence. You'll have to guide them. From here, there's a variety of things you can do. First off, you've got the insurgent on the roof over there. The insurgents just pop up. You have to learn where they are, too."

The therapist looked over Rizzo's shoulder while he brought a Black Hawk helicopter in for a flyover and then blew up another car on the street. "One thing I have to be careful about is not hitting something by accident," she said. "One time, I mistakenly clicked my mouse and all of a sudden a bullet came flying out, and I had to tell the patient that I was sorry and didn't mean to do that."

The first time I put on a head-mounted display and head-phones and entered Virtual Iraq had been in this same room, at Walter Reed, a few months earlier, after Rizzo presented prelimi-nary results from a study site to a small gathering of military officials. Rizzo was having trouble linking his laptop's PowerPoint presentation to the Walter Reed audiovisual system, and he had to speak without notes, often from a crouch behind the podium as he picked through a jumble of cables searching for one that was live. "The last one hundred years, we've studied psychology in the real world," Rizzo told the group. "In the next hundred, we're going to study it in the virtual world." He threw out some numbers. Of the five subjects who had completed treatment, four no longer met the diagnostic criteria for P.T.S.D. A fifth soldier showed no gain. (To these he would add, a few months later, the results for ten others, eight of whom had got better. Of the six research sites, San Diego was the first to have preliminary results.) After talking more generally about the features of Virtual Iraq, Rizzo invited everyone present to the fourth-floor psychiatric wing to try it out.

Although I had seen Virtual Iraq in one dimension on a computer monitor, encountering it in three dimensions, with my eyes blinkered by the headset and my ears getting a direct audio feed, was different. It still felt like make-believe, but I was fully engaged. Rizzo placed a dummy M4 rifle in my hands, and guided my fingers to a video controller fixed to the barrel. (By design, patients who use Virtual Iraq do not fire weapons; the M4 is a mood-setting device, for verisimilitude.) One toggle moved me forward, another moved me back, and a third sped me up or slowed me down. Because the display tracked with the orientation of my head, whichever way I moved determined not only what I saw but where I went. I pressed the forward button and strolled down the market street and, at Rizzo's instruction, turned at a doorway and entered a house. Inside were two insurgents, one on his knees, with his hands tied behind his back, the other dead on the ground. A baby was crying. I moved on.

The next time I put on the headset was in Marina del Rey, California, at an Institute for Creative Technologies lab space called FlatWorld, most of which was given over to life-size "mixed reality" worlds that could be negotiated without special equipment. (It was so realistic that when a virtual insurgent popped up across the virtual street from the virtual building in which I was standing, his bullets made successive holes in the virtual wall behind me and seemed to shower plaster dust through the air.) The Virtual Iraq design team, two artists and a programmer, worked out of FlatWorld, and it was their system, with the most recent improvements and additions, that I was using. This time, Rizzo sat me in a chair placed over a bass shaker, which is also known as a tactile transducer, a device that transmits the feel of sound. I slipped on the display and the headphones, and Rizzo pressed some keys on his computer and made me the driver of a Humvee, with a soldier in desert fatigues sitting next to me and another in the back. (Because the gunner was in the turret, when I looked in the rearview mirror I saw only his boots and his pant legs.) As soon as I started up the vehicle, the floor under me began to vibrate and my ears filled with the hum of tires on pavement. Suddenly, a gunman appeared on the overpass above me and started to shoot. Off to my right, a car burst into flames. Half a second later, the explosion entered my body through my feet and ears. It was startling, the way any unexpected loud noise is, but it wasn't frightening. Even when the guy in the seat next to me was shot, and his shirt sprouted a red bloom, it wasn't frightening. I had never been to Iraq. I had never been to war. The scene did not conjure any memories for me, traumatic or otherwise. It was, as JoAnn Difede said of stairs on September 10th to a person who worked in the World Trade Center, neutral.

I had seen, though, what might happen if it triggered an emotional response, when an actor named Ed Aristone, who had been cast in a movie about the Iraq conflict and wanted to get a sense of what combat was like, put on the head-mounted display at FlatWorld and found himself in the midst of a war. Rizzo cued up car bombs, shouting soldiers, ambient city sounds, blinding smoke, inert bloody bodies, the call to prayer, a child running across the street, the cough of an AK-47, snipers, a nighttime

gale—all ten plagues and their cousins at once. Aristone started
to sweat. His heart was racing. His hands were numb. He was
having a hard time holding the rifle. His face went white. He bit
his lips. After ten minutes, he said he'd had enough.

"This shows you why you need a trained therapist," Rizzo
said, turning off the machine and watching Aristone, who was
bent over, with his hands on his knees, taking deep breaths.
"Someone who knows exposure therapy, who knows how little
things can set people off. You have to understand the patient.
You have to know which stimuli to select. You'd never do what
I just did—you'd never flood them. You have to know when to
ramp up the challenges. Someone comes in and all they can do
is sit in the Humvee, maybe with the sound of wind, and may
have to spend a session or two just in that position. For P.T.S.D.,
it's really intuitive. We provide a lot of options and put them into
the hands of the clinician."

One of these is Karen Perlman, a civilian psychologist who
uses Virtual Iraq with patients at the Naval Medical Center San
Diego. Perlman is an apple-cheeked, middle-aged native Cali-
fornian with cascading brown hair, who, when I met her, was
wearing an elegant short black dress with a pink-blue-and-purple
tie-dyed silk scarf. At first glance, Perlman does not seem to be
the sort of person a young marine would cotton to, but Rizzo
says that she has a gift, and so far eight of the nine patients she
has treated no longer meet the criteria for P.T.S.D. (This number
does not account for those who dropped out.) "It's a very collab-
orative relationship," she told me in February, when Skip Rizzo
and I drove down to San Diego. "I know which stimuli I'm going
to add as the therapy progresses. I'm not going to overwhelm
them. There are no surprises. I say, 'I think you're ready for the
I.E.D. blast or for more airplanes.' I'm not only adding more,
but increasing the duration of each one. It's intensive, but for
P.T.S.D. you need a treatment that is intensive."

Although Perlman had been a clinician for more than twenty
years, before she began work with marines at the Naval Medical

Center she had never used prolonged-exposure therapy with patients, and she was surprised by its therapeutic power. (She had spent four days in Philadelphia being trained by Edna Foa, the director of the Center for the Treatment and Study of Anxiety at the University of Pennsylvania, who initially developed the prolonged-exposure technique while treating rape victims, and a day with JoAnn Difede, learning how to integrate virtual reality with exposure therapy.) "I've seen patients recover in five to six weeks," she said. "To see someone respond in such a dramatic way is very gratifying. What we're doing is very structured and systematic. It treats the core fear, the avoidance and the anxiety that are part of P.T.S.D., in a potent way. V.R. augments the therapeutic process. When the patients start to see results, usually by the fifth session, they turn the corner and get motivated."

Outside his therapist's office, Travis Boyd had "homework." He had been told to listen to an audiotape of the previous session, and to do the very things he had been avoiding—going to the mall, driving a car, calling his family back home and telling them what was really going on with him and answering their questions. He also called every one of the men who had been on the roof that day and asked them to tell him their recollections. He was surprised to learn that not one of them thought, as he had for so long, that he was responsible for their team leader's death. In fact, as they remembered it, the man had told Boyd to wait at the top of the stairs. "I had been walking around with all this guilt about getting my brother killed," Boyd said. "It just weighs on you. He was not the only friend I lost, but I was closest to him. Everyone thought it was awful that he died, but nobody thought it was my fault."

The first thing Boyd noticed, after a few weeks of Virtual Iraq exposure therapy, was that he was able to sleep without medication. He was more relaxed, and he could joke around. "Before, I felt like there were two people in me," Boyd said. "The marine, who was numb, who was a tough guy, and the civilian me, the real me, the guy who isn't serious all the time, the guy who can take a joke. By the end of therapy I felt more like one person. Toward the end, it was pretty easy to talk about what had happened over there. We went over all the hot spots in succession. I could talk about it without breaking down. I wasn't holding anything back. I felt like the weight of the world had been lifted. I was ready to be done. The last two sessions, I didn't think I needed to be there anymore."

The last time I talked to Travis Boyd, it was his third wedding anniversary. Boyd is now twenty-two, and works for a commercial construction firm in the Midwestern town where he grew up. "Most of the intrusive thoughts have gone away," he said. "You never really get rid of P.T.S.D., but you learn to live with it. I had pictures of my team leader that I couldn't look at for three years. They're up on my wall now."

Permissions

"Fixing Mr. Fix-it," by Diane Suchetka. Copyright © 2008 by Plain Dealer Publishing Co. All rights reserved. Used by permission of *The Plain Dealer*.

"A Summer of Madness" by Oliver Sacks, originally published in *The New York Review of Books*. Copyright © 2008 by Oliver Sacks, reprinted with permission of THE WYLIE AGENCY, LLC.

"Contagious Cancer," by David Quammen. Copyright © by *Harper's Magazine*. All rights reserved. Reproduced from the April issue by special permission.

"DNA Pollution May be Spawning Killer Microbes," by Jessica Snyder Sachs. Copyright © 2008 by Jessica Snyder Sachs. Reprinted by permission. As first appeared in *Discover* magazine. Jessica Snyder Sachs is the author of *Good Germs, Bad Germs: Health and Survival in a Bacterial World* (FSG/Hill & Wang).

"Real Men Get Prostate Cancer," by Dana Jennings. From *The New York Times*, November 18 © 2008. All rights reserved. Used by permission and protected by the Copyright Laws of the United States. The printing, copying, redistribution, or retransmission of the Material without express written permission is prohibited.

"I Want My Life Back," by Andrea Coller. Copyright © by Andrea Coller. Reprinted by permission. First published in *Glamour*.

"Going Under," by Jason Zengerle. Reprinted by permission of The *New Republic*, © 2009, TNR II, LLC.

"Superbugs," by Jerome Groopman. Copyright © 2008 by Jerome Groopman. Originally published by *The New Yorker*, August 2008. Reprinted by permission of William Morris Endeavor Entertainment, LLC on behalf of the author.

"Doctors Within Borders," by Susanna Schrobsdorff. Copyright © 2008 by Susanna Schrobsdorff. Reprinted by permission. First published as a *Newsweek Web Exclusive*.

"We Fought Cancer...And Cancer Won," by Sharon Begley. Copyright © 2008 by Sharon Begley. Reprinted by permission. First published in *Newsweek*.

"Duality," by Julie R. Rosenbaum. Copyrighted and published by Project HOPE/*Health Affairs* as "Duality" by Julie R. Rosenbaum, *Health Affairs*, Vol. 27, Number 2, March/April 2008, pages 494-499. The published article is available online at www.healthaffairs.org.